Eye Movements

ARVO Symposium 1976

Eye Movements

ARVO Symposium 1976

Edited by
Barbara A. Brooks
and
Frank J. Bajandas

The University of Texas Health Science Center
at San Antonio

PLENUM PRESS · NEW YORK AND LONDON

ISBN-13: 978-1-4684-2426-3   e-ISBN-13: 978-1-4684-2424-9
DOI: 10.1007/978-1-4684-2424-9

Proceedings of a Symposium on Eye Movements held at the University of Texas
Health Science Center in San Antonio, Texas, October 29-30, 1976

FOREWORD

The nature, control, and disorders of eye movements are
topics which draw together scientists from many diverse fields.
On October 29-30, 1976, a Symposium on Eye Movements was held at
The University of Texas Health Science Center at San Antonio. The
Symposium constituted the Southern Sectional Meeting of the
Association for Research in Vision and Ophthalmology. The Program
Coordinators, Drs. Frank Bajandas and Barbara Brooks invited an
outstanding group of participants to give presentations on a
variety of aspects of this subject.

This volume contains all of the invited presentations delivered
at that meeting. It does not include the excellent free papers,
nor the enthusiastic and fruitful discussions that the participants
and the audience enjoyed as well.

The editorial work for this book was performed by Dr. Brooks
and Dr. Bajandas with great care and efficiency. They have made
special efforts together with the Publisher, Plenum Press, to
bring this information to you in the shortest possible time, so as
to retain the currency of its contents.

This effort would not have been even considered without the
tireless and always dependable assistance of Mrs. Catherine Arocha
and Mrs. Louise Whelan. We are also indebted to the Texas State
Commission for the Blind for its help in defraying the expenses
ever attendant at significant symposia.

George W. Weinstein, M.D.
Professor and Head
Division of Ophthalmology
The University of Texas
Health Science Center at
San Antonio

v

CONTENTS

ENIGMAS AND HYPOTHESES...1
  David G. Cogan

DISORDERS OF EYE-HEAD COORDINATION...............................9
  David S. Zee

THE OCULAR MOTOR SYSTEM: NORMAL AND CLINICAL STUDIES...........41
  Louis F. Dell'Osso and B. Todd Troost

IS THE CEREBELLUM TOO OLD TO LEARN?............................65
  D. A. Robinson

THE PRIMATE FLOCCULUS AND EYE-HEAD COORDINATION...............75
  F. A. Miles

OPTOKINETIC NYSTAGMUS AND AFTER-NYSTAGMUS:
CHARACTERISTICS AND FUNCTIONAL SIGNIFICANCE...................93
  Bernard Cohen, Victor Matsuo and Theodore Raphan

THE ROLE OF THE BRAIN-STEM RETICULAR FORMATION IN
EYE MOVEMENT CONTROL...105
  Edward L. Keller

ABDUCENS TO MEDIAL RECTUS PATHWAY IN THE MLF:
A POSSIBLE CELLULAR BASIS FOR THE SYNDROME OF
INTERNUCLEAR OPHTHALMOPLEGIA.................................127
  Stephen M. Highstein

THE NUCLEUS PREPOSITUS HYPOGLOSSI............................145
  Robert Baker

THE NEURAL CONTROL OF SACCADIC EYE MOVEMENTS:
THE ROLE OF THE SUPERIOR COLLICULUS.........................179
  David L. Sparks and Jay G. Pollack

INDEX 221

ENIGMAS AND HYPOTHESES

David G. Cogan

Clinical Branch, National Eye Institute, National
Institutes of Health, Department of Health, Education
and Welfare, 9000 Rockville Pike, Bethesda, Maryland

A symposium embracing the basic and clinical sciences is
successful insofar as it establishes a dialogue among persons of
diverse interests and experience. We have much to give each other
but, immersed in our special disciplines and peculiar jargons, we
are prone to go our separate ways with progressive lack of inter-
communication.

As the introductory speaker in this symposium I shall present
a few clinical entities which seem to me enigmatic. Most of these
will be in the area of nystagmus. I would hope that the neuro-
physiologists here present might give some thought to our perplexities and possibly offer suggestions that are more adequate
than our present hypotheses.

1. The first example is what I have chosen to call the
sensory type of congenital nystagmus (1). This consists of
horizontal oscillations of the eyes occurring in persons who have
had bilaterally poor vision since early life. The poor vision may
have been due to retinal disease, optic atrophy, or opacities of
the media but must have dated from infancy or early childhood. In
some positions of gaze the ocular excursions are symmetric to the
two sides whence it has been designated pendular nystagmus but on
eccentric gaze the nystagmus usually becomes a jerk type with a
fast and slow component. When the visual defect is severe the
movements may be totally erratic.

A lack of retinal feed-back to stabilize the eyes has been
suggested to account for the nystagmus. But it is enigmatic that
the nystagmus occurs only when the visual failure dates from early
life. What is it about the brain which, after infancy, compensates

1

for the lack of retinal feed-back? An explanation for this age-
dependent discrepancy might bear significantly on other phenomena
of the central nervous system which show variable effects with
age.

      2. Corollary to the foregoing is the difference in the
nystagmus of the blind human infant as compared with the blind
monkey. Human beings blinded from early life develop, almost
without exception, a horizontal, predominately pendular nystagmus
whereas blinded monkeys develop a vertical, down-beat nystagmus
(2,2a). The nystagmus of blind monkeys simulates what one sees in
human beings with posterior brain-stem lesions.

      The difference between man and monkey may be related to the
directional predominance of normal eye movements in the two
species. Man's normal ocular excursions are predominately horizontal whereas the monkey's customary movements are as much
vertical as horizontal. Yet this is not an explanation and the
difference between man and monkey's response to sensory deprivation
needs clarification.

      3. A further enigmatic corollary is the vertical oscillation
of a monocularly blind eye (in human beings) of congenital origin
whereas, as noted, the oscillations are horizontal for binocularly
blind eyes. This is a rare occurrence but occurs sufficiently
frequently to constitute an established phenomenon and is, so far
as I am aware, totally unexplained.

      4. Latent nystagmus presents an enigma that also lacks a
convincing explanation. The phenomenon is congenital and consists
of a horizontal jerk-like nystagmus that is elicited by occluding
either eye. The cycle comprises a slow component toward the side
of the covered eye and a corrective saccade toward the side of the
fixing eye. While invariably bilateral and symmetric in the two
eyes it may be coarser in the presence of strabismus when the
amblyopic eye is used for fixation. Since it is not present with
strabismus until one eye is occluded and since it is not induced
in persons with binocular vision by insertion of vertical prisms,
it's pathogenesis depends on something other than simple disruption
of binocular vision. Some evidence suggests a difference in light
intensity between the two eyes is a significant factor. Pro-
gressively decreasing the light entering one eye by means of a
photographic wedge results in a progressive increase in the
amplitude of the nystagmus.

      Latent nystagmus may be the sole abnormality in the eyes and
certainly does not depend on any sensory defect. On the other
hand it is significantly often associated with the motor type of
congenital nystagmus (1).

Persons with latent nystagmus seem to have a photic tonus coming from the retina of each eye tending to turn the eyes conjugately to the opposite side. With both eyes open and equally stimulated the tonic effects are in balance and the eyes are stationary but disruption of this balance results in the nystagmus. While theoretically plausible this explanation is without experimental support and offers no accounting for its exclusive occurrence in these particular patients.

5. Spasmus nutans is a further enigma in the field of nystagmus. This abnormality consists of fine and rapid horizontal oscillations of one eye, occasionally of both eyes, occurring temporarily in some infants. The nystagmus is pendular and usually enhanced by gaze in one direction. It derives its name, unwisely, from a head nodding that may or may not be associated with it.

There is no adequate explanation for spasmus nutans although an ancient belief postulated a relationship to the rearing of infants under conditions of poor illumination. A more acceptable explanation is that it represents a delay in myelination or in neuronal assignment in the developing nervous system but there is no evidence to support this assumption either. Whatever the explanation, typical spasmus nutans is usually self-corrective after a few months and is not known to cause any significant impairment of visual functions (3).

6. Periodic alternating nystagmus is a jerk type of eye movements with a regular rhythm of 1½ - 2 minutes beating in one direction followed by a relative arrest of the eyes (or pendular oscillations) for ½ - 1 minute and then beating in the opposite direction for 1½ - 2 minutes (4). This is the typical cycle but the beating may be asymmetric and one variation consists of cyclic alternating deviation of the eyes to either side with consequent cyclic head turning (5,6).

Periodic alternating nystagmus may be a congenital occurrence but more often it occurs with lesions in the posterior fossa (7,8). The site of the responsible lesions has not been well identified.

It has been suggested that this anomaly is due to an alternating tonus of the horizontal conjugate control to the two sides but the reasons for this alternation are obscure. To my knowledge no other rhythm in the nervous system corresponds to the approximate 2-1-2 minute periodicity of this nystagmus.

7. The ophthalmoplegia of myasthenia gravis presents several enigmas. One is the selective involvement of particular eye muscles. With a systemic disease due, as currently conceived,

to a circulating inhibitor of the myoneural junction, one would
expect a uniform reduction in all eye muscle functions, as is
indeed the rule with skeletal muscles elsewhere. But in the eyes
the rule is to have individual muscles involved. The two eyes are
usually affected asymmetrically. For instance, unilateral or
asymmetric ptosis and asymmetric paralysis of only one or two
muscles is the rule in early cases. With relapses of the ophthalmoplegia the same muscles or different muscles may be involved.
The reasons for this unpredictable performance are unknown.

A further curiosity in connection with myasthenic ophthalmoplegia is a retention or even enhancement of the saccadic velocity
despite the paralysis. One would expect a slowing of eye movements
to result from the cholinergic block. Such has been reported to
be the case (9) but several of us have independently observed
normal or even hypernormal velocity in some cases of myasthenia
(10, 11, 12, 13) with, frequently, a dysmetric overshoot of the
eyes. In the case of severe ophthalmoplegia these rapid saccades
produce a twitch or quiver. Such movements are not known to occur
in myasthenic skeletal muscles elsewhere nor in other forms of
ophthalmoplegia.

Hypotheses to account for this paradoxic behavior are not
lacking. The possibility which we have favored is that the two
myoneural junction systems (the pulse and the step) which are
peculiar to eye muscles are affected to different degrees in these
patients. Both systems are known to be cholinergic but not
necessarily equally affected in myasthenia gravis. It is con-
ceivable that in the patients with twitch movements the myoneural
system responsible for initiating the saccade (the pulse) is less
affected than that system responsible for completing the saccade
and for maintaining eccentric gaze (the step). In attempting to
execute a change in fixation the patient would then generate a
saccade of normal velocity (or in the presence of an ophthalmoplegia a velocity greater than normal for the actual excursion)
but would be unable to complete the intended movement nor to hold
the gaze to one side. The result is a high-velocity, low-amplitude
movement with an apparent overshoot. It must be admitted, however,
that there is no substantive evidence either for or against this
speculation.

An alternative explanation is that momentary arrest of the
eyes in one position allows restoration of the cholinergic mediator
so that the subsequent attempt to move the eyes in the opposite
direction permits a transient burst of impulses to reach the
muscle. A similar explanation has been invoked to account for the
lid twitch in myasthenia gravis. Again there is no evidence for
or against such a hypothesis.

8. Abnormalities of the optokinetic response has posed an enigma for some of us. If the optokinetic test is a measure of the pursuit system and if each cerebral hemisphere is concerned with conjugate movements to the opposite side one would expect an abnormal response with movements of the field to the opposite side with cerebral lesions. The reverse is the case. Parietal lobe lesions result in absent or diminished response on rotation of the field to the homolateral side. Similarly paradoxic are the cog-wheel pursuit on following an object toward the side of the lesion rather than toward the opposite side and the contra-lateral deviation of the eyes toward the opposite side with closure of the lids (14). With a paresis of gaze one might expect the deviation to occur to the same side.

A possible explanation is to assume that the lesion has caused an increased tone for the conjugate gaze to the opposite side analogous to the spastic hemiplegia in the rest of the motor system. Such an explanation would account for the deviation of gaze with closure of the lids and possibly for the cog-wheel pursuit movements but less obviously for the abnormal optokinetic response.

9. Apraxia of eye movements may seem enigmatic insofar as the patient is unable to initiate conjugage gaze although the basic ocular motor mechanisms are intact. Patients with the congenital variety are unable to turn their eyes readily on command in a horizontal direction and yet move them normally at random and can execute normal vertical movements voluntarily. Also absent is the fast component of vestibular nystagmus. If the patients with congenital apraxia of conjugate gaze are asked to look to one side they will turn their head and in doing so develop a contraversive deviation of the eyes because of the vestibular input. Thus, in order to fix an object the patient will be forced to over-shoot with his head giving rise to the characteristic head thrust of this syndrome.

The acquired form of ocular motor apraxia (called Balint's syndrome) differs from the congenital variety in that the head movements are also apractic so that the compensatory head thrusts are lacking and vertical movements are involved along with the horizontal movements.

The lesion or lesions responsible for the acquired form are biparietal or fronto-parietal but there is no indication where the lesions are that are responsible for the congenital variety.

Ocular motor apraxia, like that of apraxia of other motor systems, is enigmatic only insofar as we are ignorant of the higher centers for voluntary control. In the case of congenital ocular motor apraxia there is a delay in initiation of the movement

but the movement itself has normal velocity when executed. The
assumption is that there is impairment of the higher centers, or
in Mountcastle's term, of the "get-ready" centers (15).

In conclusion, enigmas simply reflect our ignorance. The
present list comprises a small sample of what has raised questions
in my mind. The list could be extended indefinitely and I am
sure each of us would have a different order of priority. Meetings
such as this symposium offer the greatest opportunity for de-
enigmatizing problems or, at least, of sharing the perplexities
with kindred spirits.

REFERENCES

1. Cogan, D.G. Congenital nystagmus. *Canad. J. of Ophthal.*,
    2:4-10, 1967.

2. Doty, R.W. Personal communication.

2a. Pasik, P., Pasik, T., & Bender, M.B. Recovery of the electro-
    oculogram after total ablation of the retina in monkeys. *E.
    E. G. Clin. Neurophysiol.*, 19:291-297, 1965.

3. Norton, E.W., Cogan, D.G. Spasmus nutans. A clinical study
    of twenty cases followed for two years or more since onset.
    Arch. Ophthal., 52:442-446, 1954.

4. Kestenbaum, A. Periodisch umschlagender Nystagmus. *Klin.
    Monats. Augenheilk.*, 84:552, 1930.

5. Goldberg. R.T., Gonzalez, C., & Breinin, G.M. Periodic
    alternating gaze deviation with dissociation of head movement.
    Arch. Ophthal., 73:324-330, 1965.

6. Robb, R.M. Periodic alternation of null point in congenital
    nystagmus. *Arch. Ophthal.*, 87:169-173, 1972.

7. Towle, P.A. Romanul, F. Periodic alternating nystagmus.
    Neurol., 20:408, 1970.

8. Keane, J.R. Periodic alternating nystagmus with downward
    beating nystagmus. *Arch. Neurol.*, 30:399, 1974.

9. Metz, H.S., Scott, A.B., & O'Meara, D.A. Saccadic eye
    movements in myasthenia gravis. *Arch. Ophthal.*, 88:9-11,
    1972.

10. Yamazaki, A., & Ishikawa, S. Chap 3. *Eye Movements, Neuro-
    ophthalmology.* (ed.) Ishikawa, S., Egaku Shoin: Tokyo,
    (Japanese), 1974.

11. Schmidt, D. Diagnostik myasthenischer Augensyndrome. *Klin.
    Monats. Augenheilk.*, 167:651-664, 1975.

12. Cogan, D.G., Yee, R.D., & Gittinger, J.W. Rapid eye movements
    in myasthenia gravis: 1. Clinical observations. *Arch.
    Ophthal.*, 94:1083-1085, 1976.

13. Yee, R.D., Cogan, D.G., Zee, D.S., Baloh, R.W., & Honrubia,
    V. Rapid eye movements in myasthenia gravis. *Arch. Ophthal.*,
    94:1465-1472, 1976.

14. Cogan, D.G. Neurologic significance of lateral conjugate
     deviation of the eyes on forced closure of the lids. *Arch.
     Ophthal.*, 39:37-42, 1948.

15. Mountcastle, V.B. The world around us: neural command
     functions for selective attention. *Neurosci. Res. Prog.
     Bull.*, 14, April 1976.

DISORDERS OF EYE-HEAD COORDINATION

David S. Zee
Departments of Neurology and Ophthalmology
School of Medicine, The Johns Hopkins University
Baltimore, Maryland

Clinically, the neuro-ophthalmologist usually assesses ocular motility by first instructing the patient to keep his head still and then examining eye movements. Of course, this technique is both useful and necessary but we usually forget that many eye movements, and especially those of large amplitudes, are naturally associated with head movements. Consequently, the neurological control signals to the neck and eye muscles frequently coincide and probably have many features -- both functional and anatomical -- in common.

To illustrate how tightly coupled these control signals can be, one should attempt to make a rapid head movement in one direction and synchronously make a saccade in the opposite direction. Saccades and head movements can be dissociated in this way but only after conscious effort. Likewise, if a normal subject in the dark is instructed to quickly move his head without consciously directing his gaze, he will nevertheless generate a large saccade synchronous with the onset of the head movement (1,2).

Because of the natural link between eye and head movements, the study of patterns of eye-head coordination in patients with neurological disorders should be of interest to both the neuro-ophthalmologist and the ocular motor physiologist. In this presentation, I will review briefly some aspects of normal eye-head coordination and its supranuclear control and then discuss several clinical problems in which abnormal patterns of eye-head coordination occur.

NORMAL EYE-HEAD COORDINATION

Unfortunately, relatively little is known about normal patterns of eye-head coordination during rapid changes of gaze. Only a few investigators have recorded and quantitatively analyzed eye and head movements during free head tracking (3-7). The accuracy of gaze shifts, the accuracy of head movements, the velocity-amplitude and duration-amplitude relationships for head movements and the responses to closely-spaced double target jumps still need to be examined in greater detail.

Unfortunately it is technically difficult to obtain accurate recordings of head position. In methods using a helmet, slippage of the head within the helmet and the inertia of the helmet itself may cause errors. In addition, problems occur with head translation, head tilt and restriction of free head movement when a mechanical linkage to the helmet is used to transduce head position. Some of these problems have been eliminated by using a photoelectric method to record helmet position (8). More sophisticated ways of recording head movement use a search coil in a magnetic field (9) or a sensitive accelerometer (10). The coil or accelerometer can be placed on a bite bar held in the subject's mouth, or affixed to the top of the head.

For our studies, Doctor Takeshi Kasai designed a relatively simple clinical method for measuring head movements (Figure 1.). A helmet (the type used by epileptic children to prevent head injuries) is packed with sponges in the inner lining to prevent slippage. The helmet is suspended from a rotatable shaft by several layers of jigsaw blades arranged as bowed leaf springs. The shaft is linked to a low torque potentiometer and aligned with the true axis of rotation of the head. This apparatus allows for translations and rotations in all planes and transduces horizontal head position over a linear range of $\pm$ 50 degrees with a sensitivity of about 1/2 degree.

Figure 2 (left) shows the response of a normal subject to a sudden, non-predictable step change in target position (called the "triggered" mode by Bizzi and co-workers; 11). The subject was placed in a dark room and instructed to quickly move both his head and eyes to the new position of the target. After the target jump, the light was briefly flashed in its new position for 200 msec, and then extinguished. One second later, it was re-illuminated. In this way, the visual-following reflexes could not contribute to image stabilization once the head began to move. Typically, after a latency of several hundred milliseconds from the target jump, the eyes began moving toward the target and 0-40 milliseconds later, the head movement followed.

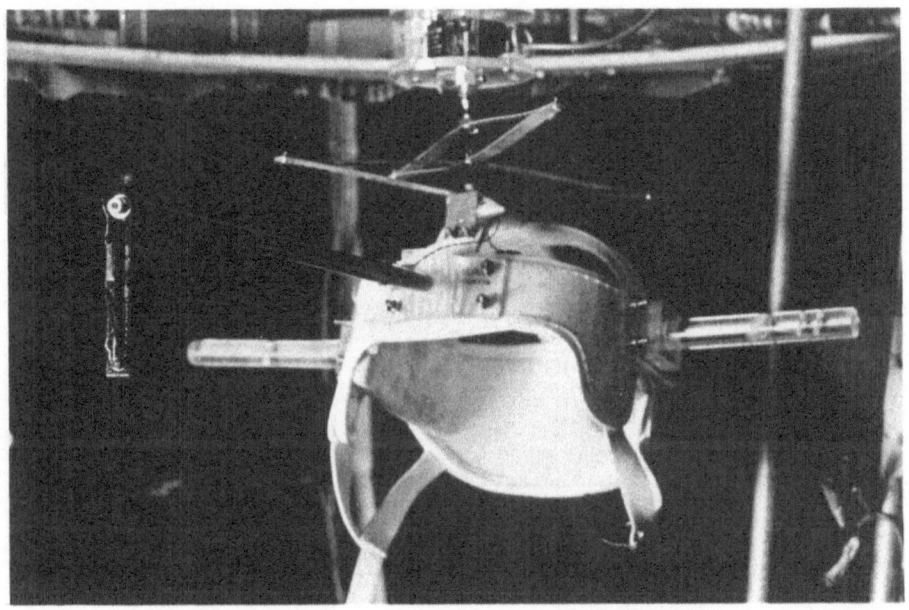

FIGURE 1. Head movement recording apparatus. Helmet is suspended
from the rotatable shaft and potentiometer by jigsaw blades
arranged as leaf springs in a bowed fashion.

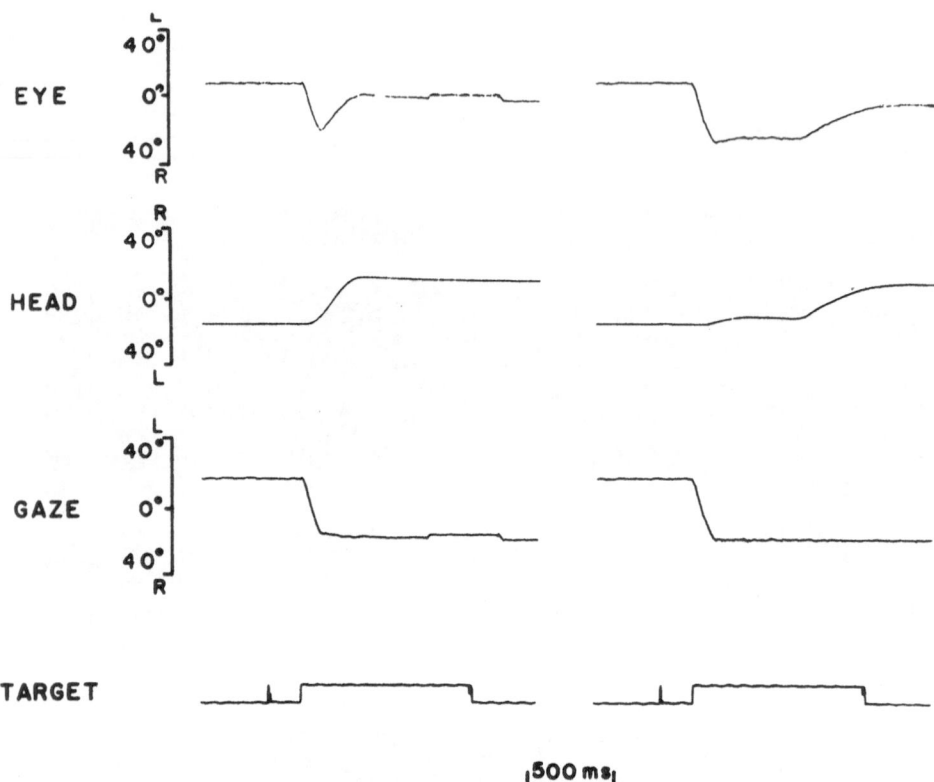

FIGURE 2. Normal eye–head coordination. EYE = Eye position in
the orbit. HEAD = Head position in space. GAZE = EYE +
HEAD = Eye position in space. Note inversion of head position
axis. Target trace shows pattern of light display. At spike,
target light jumps to new position. After 200 msec, the light
is extinguished and then re-illuminated one second later.
The pulse on the target trace indicates duration of light off.
Left: Response to non-predictable step change in target
position (36 degrees). Right: Response when the head is
blocked at onset of head movement. A normal amplitude saccade
is produced.

The movement of the eye in the orbit (EYE) reflects first the saccade alone and then, when the head begins moving, the sum of the saccade and the oppositely-directed, compensatory response which arises from the vestibulo-ocular reflex. If the head is prevented from moving just at the onset of a combined eye-head movement, a saccade is produced identical in amplitude and wave form to saccades made when the subject follows a jumping target with his head persistently immobilized (Fig 2, right). In other words, the modification of the trajectory of the saccade appears to be achieved by superposition of the neural commands from the saccadic and vestibular systems. The saccadic command is based on retinal error (the distance of an image of an object from the fovea) while the vestibular command is derived from peripheral sensory input stimulated by the head movement itself. Similar findings have been described in the monkey (12).

Meanwhile, GAZE or the position of the eye in space is the sum of the movement of the eye in the orbit (EYE) and of the head in space (HEAD) (the body is the spatial frame of reference). Since for rapid head movements the vestibulo-ocular reflex operates with a compensatory gain (eye velocity/head velocity) of unity (5, 13) the wave form of the change in gaze mirrors the wave form of a saccade made with the head immobilized. Of course, not all gaze changes are perfectly accurate or identical in wave form (see Ref. 4) just as saccades made with the head immobilized are variable. In particular, fatigue and inattention distort the response. Nevertheless, the recordings shown in Figure 2 are representative of normal behavior.

During rapid, non-predictable, passive head movements in the dark, gaze is also effectively stabilized (Figure 3). In addition, the trajectory of the quick phase of nystagmus induced by the head movement is modified by the oppositely-directly command from the vestibular system. Even during passively-induced head movements, the slow phase signal is added to the quick phase command.

Another pattern of eye-head coordination has been reported in monkeys who are trained to track a target jumping in a predictable manner (11). In this case, the head movements are less abrupt, slower, and lead the change in gaze by as much as several hundred milliseconds. We have observed a similar pattern in human beings who are tracking a target jumping in a predictable fashion or refixating between two stationary targets at a self-paced frequency (Figure 4). In this mode of eye-head coordination, too, the head movement-ocular stabilizing reflexes operate with a gain of unity and gaze is effectively stabilized.

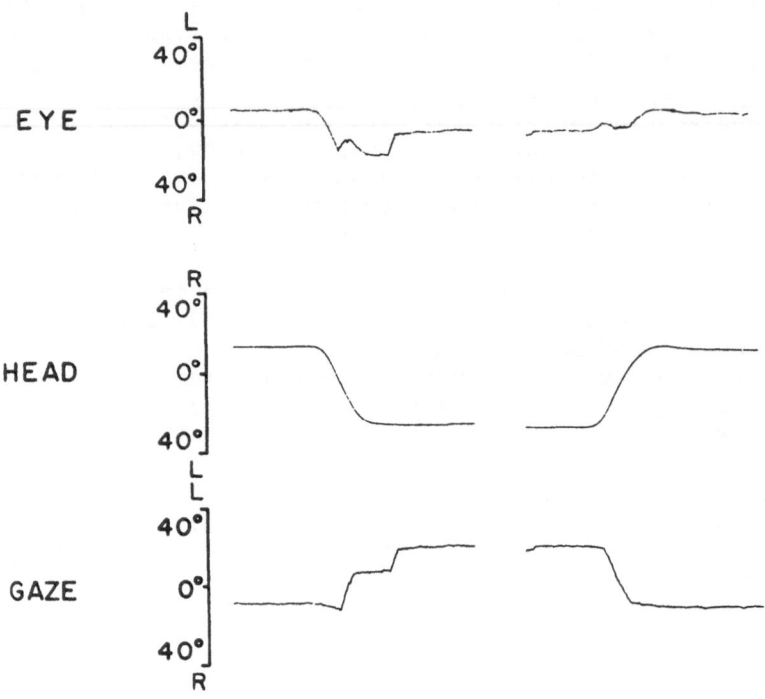

FIGURE 3. Passive, non-predictable head movement in darkness.
    Subject is performing mental arithmetic. EYE = Eye position
    in the orbit. HEAD = Head position in space. GAZE = EYE +
    HEAD = Eye position in space. Quick phase command and
    oppositely-directed vestibular command are added so that for
    high velocity head movements, eye movement in the orbit is
    minimal. However, the change in gaze mirrors the quick phase
    of command.

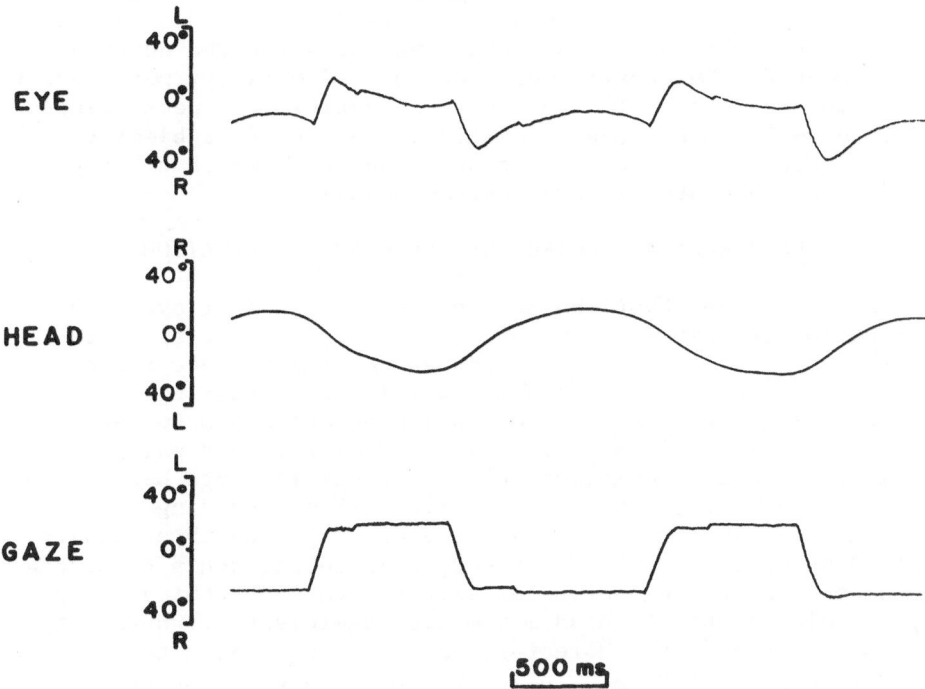

FIGURE 4. Self-paced refixations between two stationary targets
35 degrees apart. EYE = eye position in the orbit. HEAD =
Head position in space. GAZE = EYE + HEAD = Eye position in
space. Head movement leads the change in gaze.

In the monkey, the electromyographic patterns of neck muscle activity during the non-predictable "triggered" mode and the repetitive "predictable" mode are different (11). During the "triggered" mode, a brief burst of activity is recorded in the agonist coincident with silence in the antagonist. In the "predictable" mode, a smooth, reciprocal increase and decrease of activity is recorded in the agonist and antagonist.

Like saccades, it has been suggested that the rapid head movements produced during the "triggered" mode are ballistic (3, 6). In human beings, peak head velocity increases proportionately to the amplitude of the head movement while the duration of the movement remains nearly constant (3). Similarly, measurements of head movements and electromyographic activity of neck muscles in both normal and cervically deafferented monkeys subject to various inertial and constant torque loads suggest that "triggered" head movements are preprogrammed (14).

SUPRANUCLEAR CONTROL OF EYE-HEAD COORDINATION

Our knowledge about the supranuclear control of eye-head coordination is sparse. Many of the structures that are presumably important for saccades such as the frontal eye fields, superior colliculus and cerebellar vermis are either not directly concerned with head movements or show a relationship to head movements different from that to eye movements. For example, frontal eye field stimulation in monkeys elicits both head and eye movements. However, Bizzi and Schiller (15), recording from single neurons in the frontal eye fields, reported three separate populations of cells. Some discharged in relationship to saccades, others to pursuit and vestibular slow phases and a third group only in relationship to head movements regardless of whether the eye was moving or not. Moreover, the neurons related to head movements began discharging prior to the head movement while the neurons related to eye movements discharged during but not before saccades. Even so, the duration of the neural activity related to head movement was not time-locked to the duration of the head movement itself. Also bilateral frontal lobe lesions in trained monkeys apparently do not alter the animal's ability to produce either saccadic eye movements or a normal pattern of eye-head coordination (E. Bizzi, personal communication).

Stryker and Schiller (16) found that stimulation of the superior colliculus in the alert monkey elicited both head and eye movements. However, saccades were of short latency, stereo-typed, had a definite electrical threshold and were independent of the initial position of the eye in the orbit. In contrast, head movements were variable in size and latency, had no definite electrical threshold and depended on initial eye position. Head

movements were more likely to occur when the eye was contralaterally deviated in the orbit. In single unit recordings from
the intermediate layers of the superior colliculus in alert monkeys,
Robinson and Jarvis (17) found that neurons encoded eye but not
head movements.

In the brain stem, eye and head movements appear to be more
tightly coupled than in the superior colliculus or frontal eye
fields. Fuller and Miles (18) described neurons in the vestibular
nucleus that discharged in relation to both intended head movements
and eye movements. Bender and co-workers (19) and more recently
Westheimer and Blair (20) reported the patterns of eye and head
movements after brain stem stimulation in the monkey. In the
rostral tegmentum of the mesencephalon, stimulation usually
elicited ipsilateral tilt and contralateral turning of the head
while in the caudal tegmentum of the pons, stimulation caused
strong ipsilateral jerking head movements. Head movements could
occur without eye movements if the intensity of stimulation was
low. When eye and head movement occurred together, they were
usually in the same direction. Vertical head movements could only
be elicited by stimulation in the median plane and their direction
was often determined by the parameters of stimulation rather than
the location of the stimulus itself.

In the cerebellum experimental lesions indicate a dissocia-
tion between the control of head and eye movements. Ritchie (21)
showed in trained monkeys that ablation of Lobules V, VI, and VII
of the vermis caused dysmetria of saccades that depended on the
initial position of the eye in the orbit. Centering saccades were
hypermetric while eccentric saccades were hypometric. However,
during free head tracking, head movements were accurate while gaze
(which reflects the saccadic command) remained dysmetric in the
same pattern as occurred during refixations with the head immobilized.

CLINICAL DISORDERS OF EYE-HEAD COORDINATION

CEREBELLAR DISORDERS

To further study the function of the cerebellum in ocular
motor control, we have measured eye and head movements in a
patient with a vascular malformation that angiographically appeared
to involve the superior cerebellar vermis. With the head immobilized, this patient frequently made hypermetric saccades which
were especially prominent when the patient refixated toward the
primary position (Figure 5, right). During free head tracking of
a jumping target, head dysmetria was prominent with both under and
overshoots. However, in either case, the change in gaze was
usually hypometric (Figure 5). These abnormalities could be

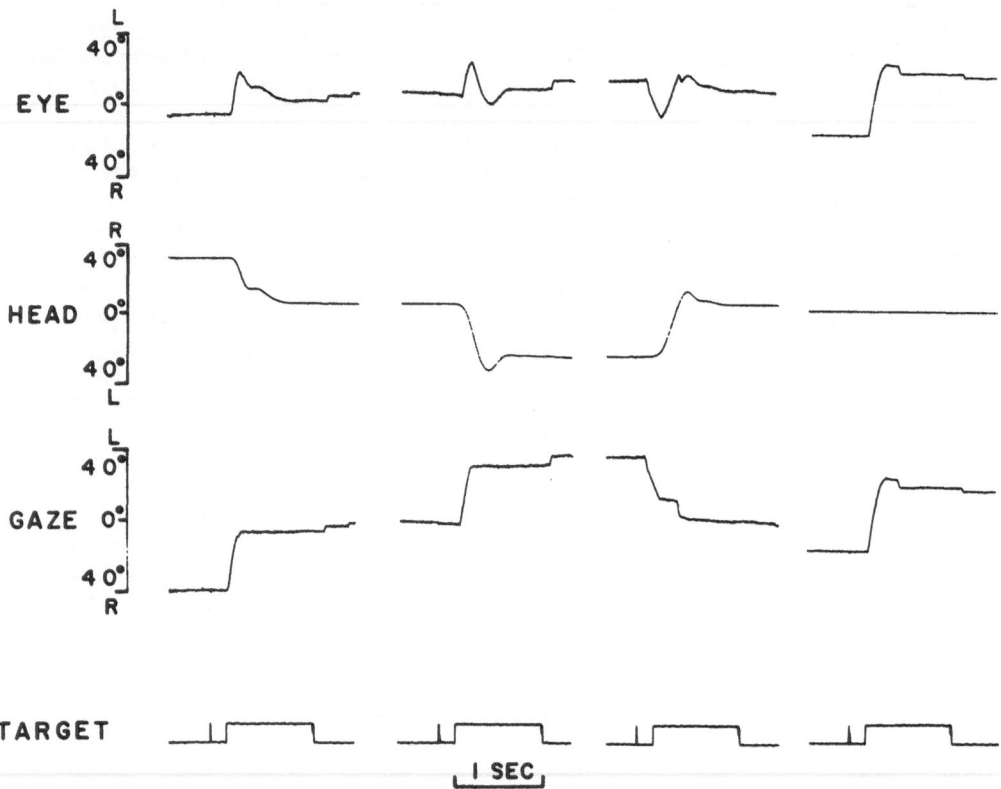

FIGURE 5. Patterns of saccadic, head, and gaze dysmetria in a
    patient with cerebellar dysfunction. EYE = Eye position in
    the orbit. HEAD = Head position in space. GAZE = EYE +
    HEAD = Eye position in space. Target trace as in Figure 2.
    Patient shows hyper- and hypometric head movements in
    association with hypometric gaze changes. With the head
    immobilized (right), saccadic hypermetria occurs.

easily observed at the bedside by instructing the patient to
rapidly move both his head and eyes between two targets.

Despite the prominence of this patient's saccadic hypermetria,
gaze overshoot was not present when his head was free to move.
This discrepancy occurred, in part, because most gaze changes
during free head tracking begin with the eyes near the primary
position in the orbit and therefore require a centrifugally-
directed saccadic command (our patient's saccadic hypermetria
usually occurred with centripetally-directed saccades). Naturally,
we infrequently make large amplitude, centripetally-directed
saccadic eye movements. Only when the neuro-ophthalmologist
immobilizes our head or perhaps when we persistently focus our
attention upon a single point in space might we make saccades of
large amplitude directed toward the primary position.

Furthermore, if the head movement-ocular stabilizing reflexes
are functioning normally with a compensatory gain of one, dysmetria
of head movements will not directly affect gaze accuracy. Even
though this patient's head often oscillated at the end of a movement, no change in gaze occurred. However, head movement amplitude
might indirectly affect the size of the change in gaze if the
program producing the neural commands for head movements can
modify, either directly or reflexively through the vestibular
system, those programs producing the neural commands for the
saccade.

CONGENITAL OCULAR MOTOR APRAXIA

Congenital ocular motor apraxia is an unusual ocular motor
disorder in which abnormal patterns of eye-head coordination
occur. Patients with this disorder cannot make normal voluntary
horizontal saccades when the head is immobilized. When the head
is free to move, they conspicuously thrust their heads. The
etiology of this syndrome is not known and pathological exami-
nations of the brains of patients with this disorder have not been
reported. The patients usually have no localizing neurological
findings.

Recently, we investigated several patients with this disorder
and found a number of ocular motor abnormalities (22). For the
saccadic system, patients showed delayed initiation (increased
latency) and marked hypometria of saccadic eye movements during
attempted refixations with the head immobilized. The degree of
abnormality was directly related to the amount of volition inherent in the visuo-motor task. For example, refixations to
verbal commands were performed less well than refixations while
tracking a jumping target. Least affected were corrective saccades
during attempted smooth pursuit tracking. Voluntary saccades made

in complete darkness were also impaired. On the other hand,
patients showed only mild abnormalities in the generation of quick
phases of optokinetic nystagmus (to full field stimulation) or
vestibular nystagmus (in response to an impulse of acceleration).

The most severely affected patient could not make a voluntary
saccade greater than 8 degrees in amplitude with his head immobilized. Latencies to the initial saccade ranged between 275-
800 milliseconds. Subsequent corrective saccades were also
hypometric and delayed. However, quick phases of optokinetic and
vestibular nystagmus were generated nearly normally and some had
amplitudes as large as 30 degrees.

This patient, despite a severe defect of voluntary saccades,
could change gaze more effectively when his head was free to move.
For example, Figure 6 shows his pattern of eye-head coordination
when he attempted to follow a 40 degree target jump. As in normal
individuals, his eyes usually slightly led the onset of the head
movement. The latency, in this case, was only 240 msecs. His
gaze change (38 degrees), which mirrored the size of the saccadic
command, was only slighly hypometric. The head movement (50
degrees) was hypermetric. However, the head overshoot itself did
not increase the amplitude of the change in gaze since the gain of
his head movement-ocular stabilizing system was one.

We next determined the relationship between the size and
velocity of head movements and the initial change in gaze. A
number of combined eye-head movements elicited in response to 20
degree target jumps were recorded. We found that both head
amplitude and head velocity were correlated with the amplitude of
the initial change in gaze. The larger and faster the head
movement, the more effectively this patient could change gaze.

These findings suggest that the thrusting, overshooting head
movements of these patients are a compensatory mechanism to help
change gaze. This facilitation is not a result of passive vestibular stimulation since the onset of the saccade usually was
synchronous with or led the onset of the head movement. Rather,
the head movement command itself, in some way, increases the
amplitude of or actually triggers the saccadic command which in
turn facilitates a change in gaze.

This patient also occasionally made head movements which
preceded the change in gaze and the pattern of rapid eye movements
resembled the quick phases of vestibular nystagmus rather than
voluntary saccades (Figure 7). We cannot prove these rapid
movements were quick phases of nystagmus. (When the head is
moving, how does one decide if a rapid movement in the direction

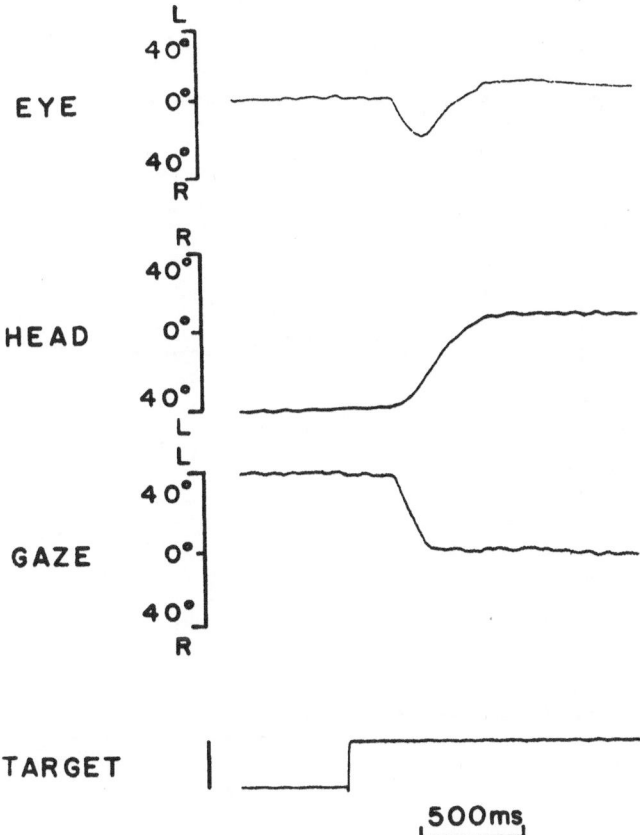

FIGURE 6. Ocular motor apraxia. Response to 40 degree target
jump (40 deg L – 0 deg). EYE = Eye position in the orbit.
HEAD = Head position in space. GAZE = EYE + HEAD = Eye
position in space. Target light is continuously illuminated.
With head free to move a large gaze change is possible. The
head movement is hypermetric.

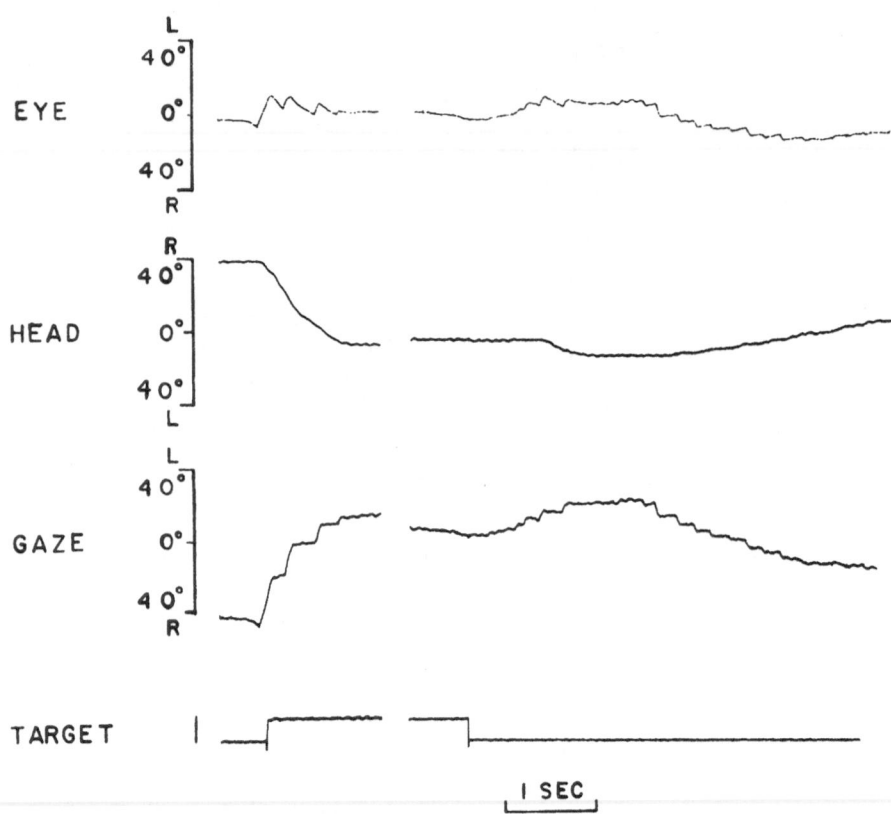

FIGURE 7. Ocular motor apraxia. Response to 40 degree target
jumps (40 deg R – 0 deg, 0 deg – 40 deg R). EYE = Eye position
in the orbit. HEAD = Head position in space. GAZE = EYE +
HEAD = Eye position in space. <u>Left</u>: Rapid head movement
which overshoots the target. Eye position trace resembles
vestibular nystagmus. <u>Right</u>: Slower head movement which
initially moves in wrong direction. Nystagmus pattern is
observed. Gaze is stable between quick phases.

of head movement is a reflexively-induced quick phase or a voluntary saccade?) However, one can hypothesize that by simply moving
his head, the patient could reflexively stimulate his intact
vestibular system to produce quick phases of nystagmus which would
in effect move the eyes in space toward the new fixation target.

To summarize, this patient used head movements to increase
the amplitude of the change in gaze by two mechanisms. First, by
making larger and faster head movements, he could indirectly
increase the size of the saccadic command which resulted in
larger gaze shifts. Secondly, he may have directly stimulated the
vestibular system to reflexively produce quick phases of nystagmus.
The use of both these strategies supports the suggestions by
Gresty (3, 23) and Barnes (2, 24) of a close relationship between
the mechanisms generating quick phases of nystagmus during passive
head movements and voluntary saccades during active head movements.

Our patient did not use another possible mechanism for
facilitating a change in gaze. He could have decreased the gain
of his vestibulo-ocular reflex. This would, of course, have
created disabling oscillopsia unless he could have learned to
suppress the vestibulo-ocular reflex selectively during active
head movements.

Patients with neurological disorders that affect both quick
phases of nystagmus and saccades (abnormally low velocities or
amplitudes or markedly increased latencies) may show still another
pattern of eye-head coordination. They may adopt the strategy of
making a rapid, large head movement which significantly overshoots
the position of the target. Through the action of the intact slow
phase of the vestibulo-ocular reflex, the eyes are brought to a
position of extreme contraversive deviation in the orbit. Then,
as the head continues moving, the eyes are carried in space to
the position of the target. The head is then rotated backward
toward the target and the eyes steadily maintain fixation of the
target as they are returned to the primary position by the action
of the vestibulo-ocular reflex. Clinically, such a pattern has
been observed in a patient who made slow saccades in association
with a spino-cerebellar degeneration (25) and also has been
reported in prior studies of some patients with ocular motor
apraxia (26).

The study of such patients illustrates that examination of
saccades alone may not reveal the true functional capacity of a
patient's ability to change gaze. When eye movements during both
passive and active head movements are also examined, a more complete
description of ocular motor function and of the adaptive strategies
used by the central nervous system to compensate for disordered
ocular motility is possible.

EYE-HEAD COORDINATION IN LABYRINTHINE-DEFECTIVE HUMAN BEINGS

The patterns of eye-head coordination in human beings with
absent labyrinthine function are of particular clinical interest
because patients with vestibular dysfunction frequently complain
of oscillopsia during head movements (27). Dichgans, Bizzi and
co-workers have previously studied head and eye movements in
bilaterally labyrinthectomized monkeys (28, 29). They discovered
three distinct compensatory mechanisms used by the labyrinthectomized monkey to recover the ability to stabilize gaze during
head movements. First, the gain of the cervico-ocular reflex was
potentiated after labyrinthectomy. In the normal monkey, the
cervico-ocular reflex contributes little to ocular stabilization
during rapid gaze shifts in the "triggered" mode (gain is less
than .05). However, in the labyrinthectomized monkey, the passively induced gain of the cervico-ocular reflex increased to
about .30, while during active movements it apparently reached
values near 0.80.

Two other compensatory phenomena were demonstrated when the
animal's head was prevented from moving just at the onset of a
"triggered" eye-head movement. First, the animal produced a
backward, slow compensatory eye movement after the saccade even
though the animal's head had never actually moved in space. In
other words, the labyrinthectomized monkey developed the ability
to preprogram compensatory eye movements during active head movements. Secondly, the amplitude of the saccade was less than that
of saccades made with the head persistently immobilized. In an
attempt to compensate for the gaze overshoot caused by the
diminished gain of the head movement-ocular stabilizing system,
the monkey recalibrated the relationship between saccadic amplitude
and retinal error selectively during active eye-head movements.

We have made preliminary observations in three adults who are
deaf and lost all vestibular function from childhood meningitis.
(T. Kasai and D. S. Zee, Eye-Head Coordination in Labyrinthine-
Defective Human Beings, in preparation). Our results are perhaps
best summarized in the last line from a delightful vignette written
about 20 years ago by a physician in New England who had permanently
lost vestibular function from streptomycin toxicity (30). After
several years, the patient had at last recovered the ability to
play tennis although he limited himself to doubles. The physician
summed up his feelings and our experimental results as follows:
"Is there any man-made machine designed like the human apparatus
with so many alternate systems to accomplish its end?"

Our patients showed no response to caloric stimulation nor
any consistent response to rotational stimuli. However, during
0.5 Hz en bloc rotation each showed an inconstant, low gain (less
than 0.15) ocular response with a large phase lead. This response

perhaps arises from skin, muscle or joint proprioceptors in the
legs or torso. Ocular nystagmus from torsion of the pelvis on the
body ("pelvic nystagmus") has been previously reported in human
beings (31).

Figures 8 and 9 show typical patterns of one of our patient's
responses to a non-predictable jumping target. The patient was
instructed to quickly move both his head and eyes to the new
position of the target. Both continuously illuminated and flashing
target (200 msecs) stimuli were used. However, each type of response
was observed in either test condition.

The initial parameters of eye-head coordination in our
patients were normal. In the continuously illuminated target
conditions, the eye and head movements began nearly synchronously
after a mean latency of 270 msec. The mean amplitude of head
movements made up about 80% of the total gaze displacement.
However, in view of the excellent compensation reported in the
labyrinthectomized monkey, this patient's ability to stabilize
gaze during head movements was surprisingly inadequate. In
Figure 8 (left), gaze drifted in the direction of head movement
because the ratio of the velocity of the compensatory eye movement
to head velocity was only 0.3. To correct gaze overshoot, the
patient made saccades in the same direction as his inadequate
compensatory eye movements. These corrective movements occurred
even when the target light had been extinguished.

Figure 8 (right) depicts another pattern of compensation.
Compensatory eye movements were transiently adequate so that gaze
was effectively stabilized in the first 50 msecs after the termination of the initial gaze change. However, the duration of this
compensatory movement was too short so that during the latter
portion of the head movement gaze drifted in the direction of head
movement. A subsequent corrective movement was necessary to
prevent gaze overshoot. In addition, the amplitude of the initial
gaze change (which nearly corresponds to the initial saccadic
command) was less than the retinal error. Presumably this represents an attempt to compensate for gaze overshoot. Nevertheless,
at times, compensation was so poor that even though the initial
saccade was small, gaze still significantly overshot the target
(Figure 9, right).

Figure 9 (left, center) shows a third type of response in
which overcompensation occurs. In this case, just after the
initial rapid gaze change, another eye movement is generated in
the direction opposite to the head movement. At times, this movement
was much faster than the head movement and appeared to be a saccade
(Figure 9, left). At other times, this movement was slow, of longer
duration and only moderately exceeded head velocity. In this

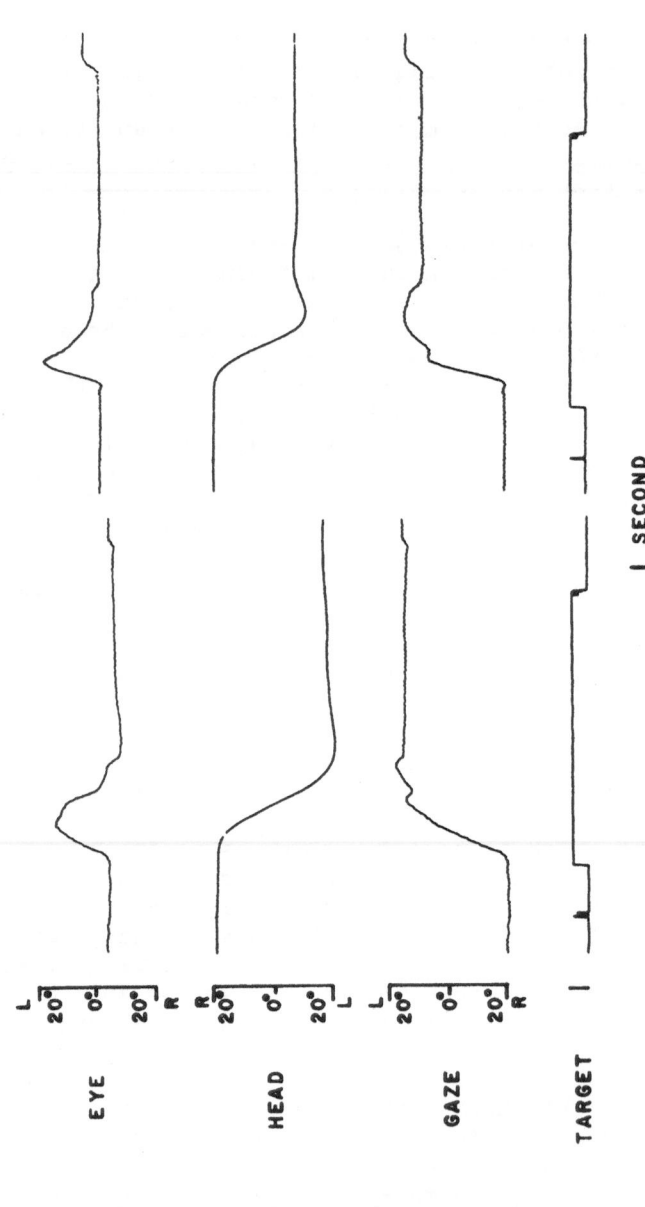

FIGURE 8. Labyrinthine-defective human response to non-predictable 38 degree target jumps. EYE = Eye position in the orbit. HEAD = Head position in space. GAZE = EYE + HEAD = Eye position in space. Target trace as in Figure 2. <u>Left</u>: Inadequate compensatory eye movements cause overshoot. <u>Right</u>: Gaze is transiently stabilized after end of initial saccade. However, before the head movement finishes, compensatory movements decrease in velocity and gaze overshoots. The amplitude of the initial rapid gaze change is hypometric.

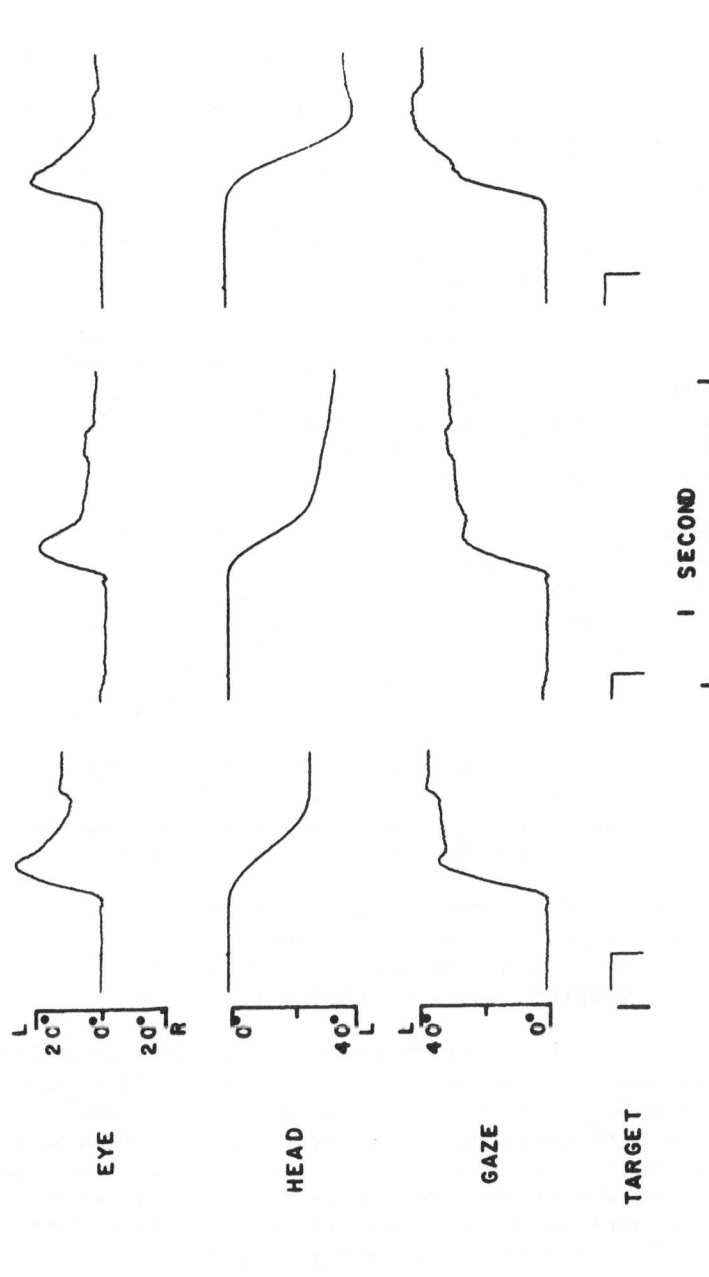

FIGURE 9. Labyrinthine-defective human response to non-predictable 38 degree target jumps. EYE = Eye position in the orbit. HEAD = Head position in space. GAZE = EYE + HEAD = Eye position in space. Target light is continuously illiminated. Left, center: Over compensation causes transient gaze undershoot by a backward saccade (left) or slower compensatory movement (center). Right: Gaze overshoot requiring backward saccade.

case, gaze drifted slowly backward (Figure 9, center). The patient occasionally showed nearly perfect gaze stability, but a normal response comprised less than 10% of all trials. However, his performance was improved when the target moved in a predictable fashion.

In order to delineate the mechanisms used by this patient to generate compensatory eye movements, we performed a blocking experiment comparable to that described by Dichgans and co-workers in the monkey (28). At the onset of a combined eye-head movement, head motion was stopped by manually immobilizing the helmet. Unfortunately, we could not totally eliminate slippage of the head within the helmet which, if it occurred, could artifactually simulate preprogramming of compensatory eye movements. In addition, at times, patients anticipated a block and purposively changed their pattern of head movement. Nevertheless, we repetitively encouraged our subjects to make a rapid head movement with each gaze change and we blocked the head as non-predictably as possible. Even so, interpretation of our findings is limited by the pitfalls of the experimental technique.

Figure 10 shows examples of blocking experiments in both the target flash and continuous target paradigms. In each case, the initial saccade is hypometric and forward corrective saccades must be made to acquire the target. In contrast, when the patient tracked targets with his head persistently immobilized, saccades were accurate.

The blocking experiments in this patient did not consistently show preprogramming of compensatory eye movement of the type described in the monkey. On a few occasions, a backward drift of maximum amplitude of about 4 degrees was observed. Slippage of the head within the helmet might have produced this result. However, even if it didn't, the amplitude of these "preprogrammed" movements was relatively small compared to the amplitude of compensatory movements actually observed during active head movements. However, in our other patients, we have more con- vincing evidence that preprogramming of this type occurs.

In order to determine the contribution of the cervico-ocular reflex to gaze stabilization, we measured rotation of the head on the body and the body on the head in the dark. Both passive and active movements were elicited. To induce active movements, the patient was instructed to move his head in approximately the same pattern as was applied during passive rotation. Patients were instructed either to perform mental arthmetic or to direct their gaze at an imagined location of a stationary target on the wall in front of them.

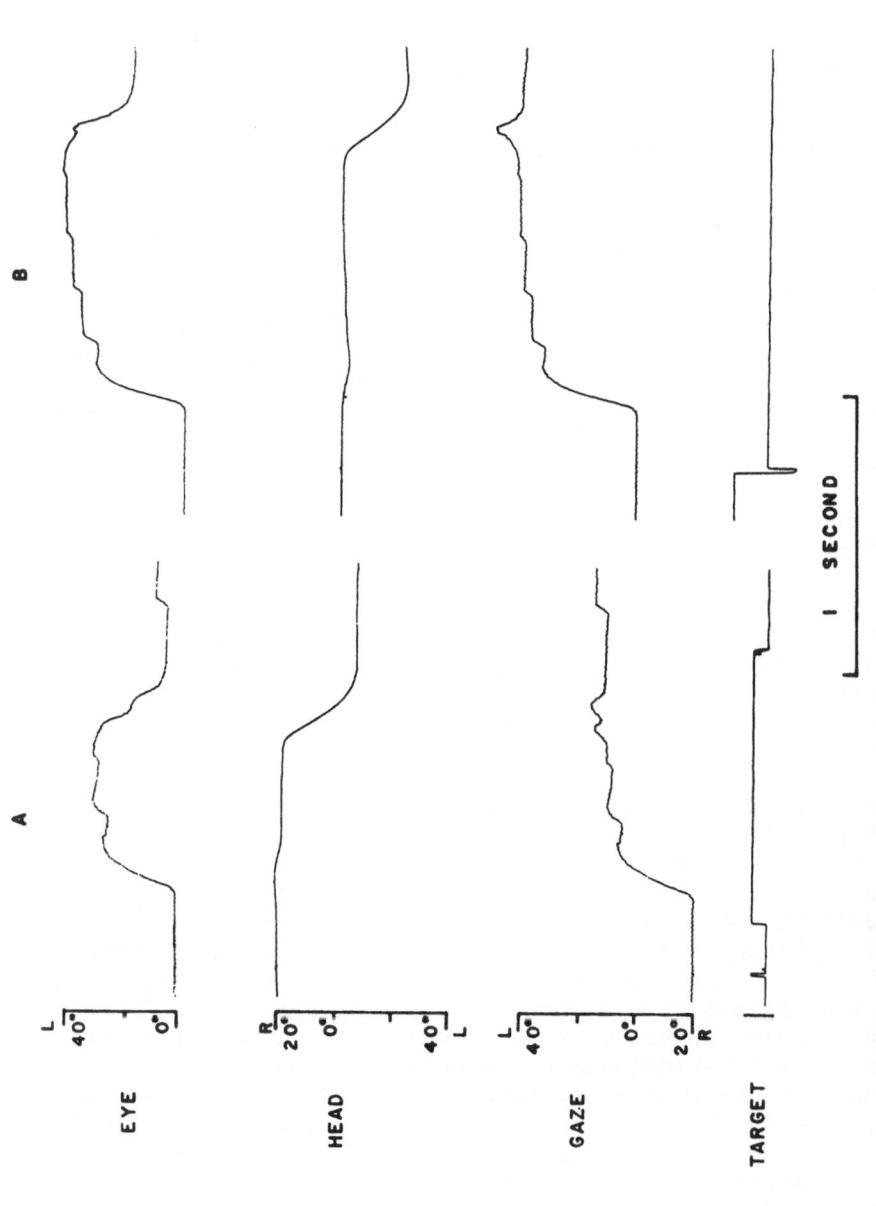

FIGURE 10. Labyrinthine-defective human being. EYE = Eye position in the orbit. HEAD = Head position in space. GAZE = EYE + HEAD = Eye position in space. Head is blocked at onset of head movement for 38 degree target jump. A. Target flash stimulus (target trace as in Figure 2). B. Target light is continuously illuminated. In both cases, the initial saccade is hypometric. Preprogrammed compensatory eye movements after the saccade are not prominent.

One methodological problem was encountered. During passive
rotation, it was difficult to rotate the subject's head in a
predictable fashion without the subject actively entraining his
head movements with the passive rotation. In particular, Patient
2 could not relax and permit exclusively passive sinusoidal
rotation of his head.

The results are summarized in the Table. We found that the
gain of the cervico-ocular reflex could be potentiated when the
patient used the effort of spatial localization to imagine a
target on the wall. The gain was also higher during active
rather than passive movements. The latter increase may also be
related to effort of spatial localization since naturally occurring
active head movements are usually related to a change of gaze to a
new point of interest in space. As indicated before, when a
normal subject is instructed to move his head in the dark without
consciously directing his gaze, he still makes a large saccade in
the direction of head movement. Therefore, it may be difficult to
eliminate the effort of spatial localization during active head
movements.

We also compared body on head rotation (neck torsion) to head
on body rotation when the patient was performing mental arithmetic
in darkness. For Patient 1, the gains were comparable. However,
Patient 2 had a lower gain during body on head rotation than
during head on body rotation. This discrepancy might be attributed
to the inability of Patient 2 to adequately relax his neck musculature during passive head rotation. For both patients, the gain
of the cervico-ocular reflex during body on head rotation decreased
with increasing frequency.

The pattern of quick phases during body on head rotation is
shown in Figure 11. For Patient 2, quick and slow phases of
nystagmus were in opposite directions. Quick phases usually took
the eye to a position in the orbit in the direction of the change
in head position relative to the position of the body. In other
words, quick phases were used to redirect gaze in the direction of
apparent head movement. On the other hand, Patient 1 usually made
quick and slow phases of nystagmus in the same direction. For
this patient, quick phases were perhaps used to correct for position
errors arising from inadequate compensatory eye movements rather
than to redirect the center of attention. During active eye-head
movements, even in the dark, this patient frequently made saccades
in the direction opposite to that of the head movement in order to
aid gaze stabilization. It is possible that this pattern of
corrective saccades during active target seeking may have become
so automatic that it occurred even when vestibular nystagmus was
induced during body on head rotation in darkness.

TABLE: CERVICO—OCULAR REFLEX (0.5 Hz)[1]

	Patient 1	Patient 2
	Gain[2]	
Head on Body		
Passive		
Mental Arithmetic	.36 ± .05[3]	.86 ± .09
Imagination	1.01 ± .26	.93 ± .07
Active		
Mental Arithmetic	.60 ± .12	.96 ± .05
Imagination	.88 ± .19	.97 ± .07
Body on Head		
Mental Arithmetic	.27 ± .10	.50 ± .14

[1]Peak—Peak Amplitude = 25-35 degrees during passive rotation and 40-50 degrees during active rotation

[2]Gain = Peak eye velocity/peak head velocity

[3]Values = Mean gain ± S.D., N ≥ 10

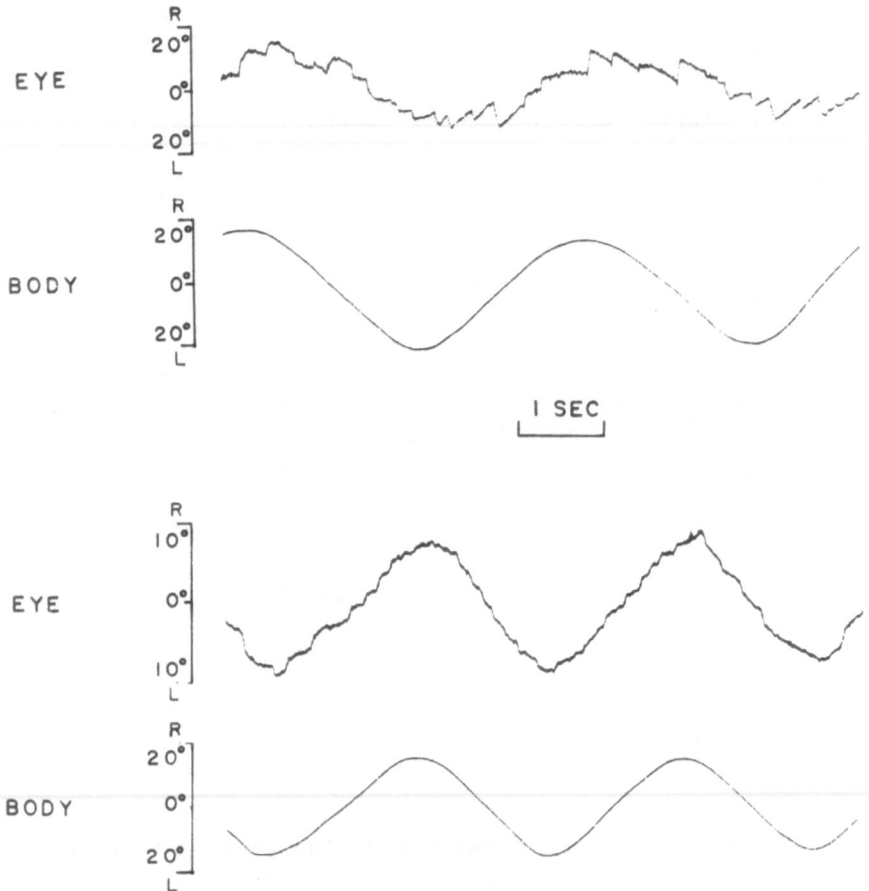

FIGURE 11. Labyrinthine-defective human being. Body on head
   rotation (head immobilized). Patients are in darkness
   performing mental arithmetic. EYE = Eye position in the
   orbit. BODY = Body position in space. Top (Patient 2):
   normal pattern of slow and quick phases of nystagmus.
   Bottom (Patient 1): Quick and slow phases of nystagmus
   occur in same direction.

To assess the contribution of the cervico-ocular reflex to gaze stabilization during active target seeking, we measured the ocular response to non-predictable, rapid, step-like head movements in the dark (Figures 12 and 13). Both passive and active head movements were elicited. To generate active head movements, patients were instructed to quickly move the head from one side to the other whenever the shoulder was tapped. Patients were instructed either to perform mental arithmetic or to continuously fixate the imagined location of a stationary target on the wall. In the passive, mental arithmetic paradigm (Figure 12, left), the gain of the cervico-ocular reflex was low (mean 0.20). The latency from neck to eye movement was long and varied between 40-100 msecs. From these two observations, we conclude that the passive, cervico-ocular reflex alone plays a minor role in stabilization of gaze during active target seeking. However, even during passive head movements with mental arithmetic, more rapid compensatory movements and even saccades oppositely directed to the head movement were occasionally observed. These compensatory movements were similar to those recorded during active target seeking.

The passive cervico-ocular reflex was significantly potentiated when the patient was instructed to hold his gaze upon an imaginary target located on the wall in front of him (Figure 12, right). With some passive head movements, the velocity of compensatory eye movements matched head velocity although their amplitudes were frequently different. Position correcting saccades were also observed.

During active rotation in the dark while performing mental arithmetic (Figure 13, left), a saccade was generated synchronously with the head movement. Gaze stability was not perfect but better than during the passive, mental arithmetic paradigm.

Finally, during active head movements with imagination of a target (Figure 13, right), the initial saccade was suppressed and gaze stabilization was most effective. The velocity of compensatory eye movements usually matched head velocity.

In summary:

1. Compensation for lost peripheral labyrinthine function is reasonably adequate but, at least for one patient, not as complete as that reported for the monkey.

2. The passive, cervico-ocular reflex makes a small contribution to gaze stability during rapid head movements.

PASSIVE

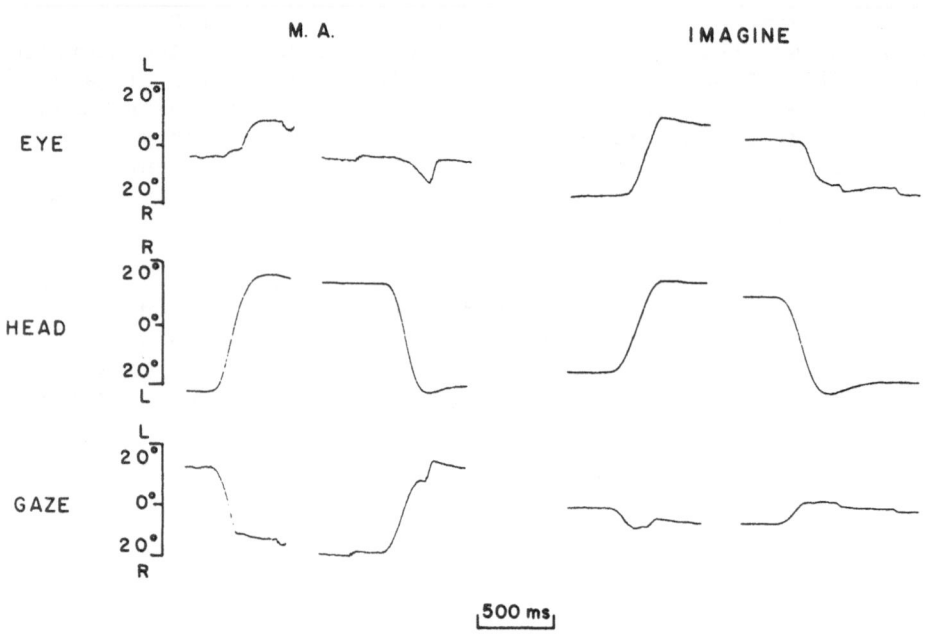

FIGURE 12. Labyrinthine-defective human being. Passive, non-
predictable, head rotations in darkness. EYE = Eye position
in the orbit. HEAD = Head position in space. GAZE = EYE +
HEAD = Eye position in space. With mental arithmetic (M.A.),
the gain (peak eye velocity/peak head velocity) of the cervico-
ocular reflex is low although occasionally higher velocity
compensatory movements are seen. With imagination of a target
on the wall (IMAGINE), the gain is often near one although
amplitude mismatches may occur.

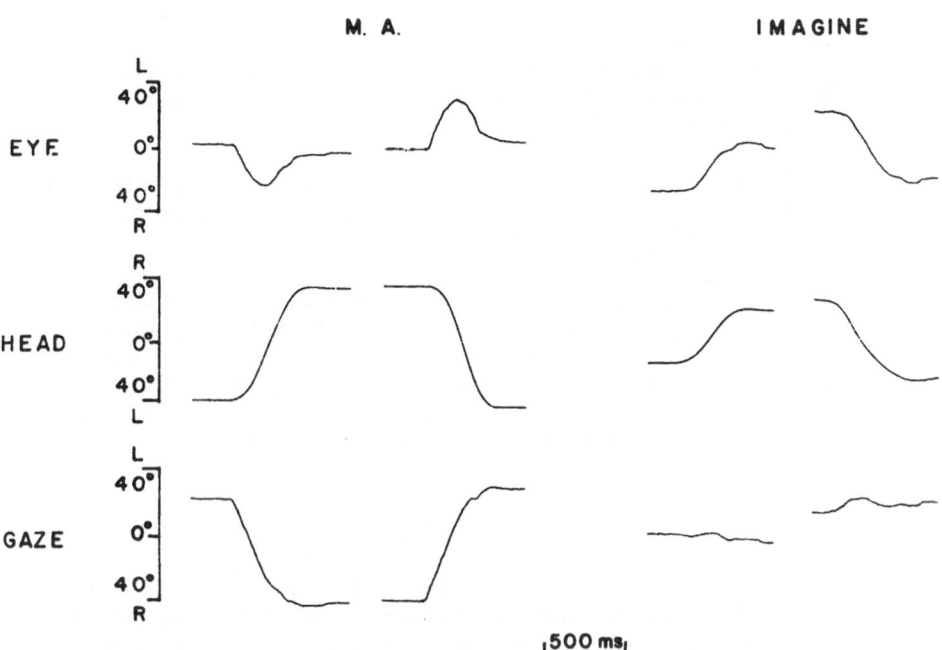

FIGURE 13. Labyrinthine-defective human being. Active-head
rotations in darkness. EYE = Eye position in the orbit.
HEAD = Head position in space. GAZE = EYE + HEAD = Eye
position in space. With mental arithmetic (M.A.), a saccade
is usually initiated synchronously with the onset of head
movement. Gaze stability is only moderately effective. With
imagination of a target on the wall (IMAGINE), the initial
saccade is suppressed and gaze stability is nearly perfect.

3.   A number of strategies are used to improve gaze stability
     including corrective saccades, slower compensatory
     movements and recalibration of the relationship between
     saccadic amplitude and retinal error during active
     target seeking.

4.   Preprogramming of compensatory eye movements of the type
     described during blocking experiments in labyrinthec-
     tomized monkeys makes a variable contribution to gaze
     stability. Patients also appear to generate compensatory
     eye movements which require an actual head movement for
     their occurrence. However, the duration of these eye
     movements were not necessarily time-locked to the
     duration of the head movement and velocity mismatches
     were frequent.

5.   Both the effort of spatial localization and predictive
     mechanisms play important roles in determining the
     adequacy of gaze stability.

6.   One of our patients showed an abnormal quick phase
     mechanism of vestibular nystagmus during body on head
     rotation. Quick phases were made in the wrong direction,
     i.e. in the _same_ direction as compensatory slow phases.
     This pattern of nystagmus may reflect an attempt to use
     quick phases to help stabilize gaze rather than redirect
     the center of attention.

ACKNOWLEDGEMENTS

    Dr. Takeshi Kasai participated in most of the investigations
described in this presentation and designed and constructed the
head position monitor. Miss Vendetta Matthews provided editorial
assistance. This work was supported by a Teacher Investigator
Award (5 K07 NS11071-02) and Research Grant (1 R01 EY01849-0)
from the National Institutes of Health.

REFERENCES

1. Henriksson, N.G., Novotny, M., and Tjernstrom, O.   Eye movements as a function of active headturnings. *Acta Oto-laryngol.*, 77:86-91, 1974.

2. Barnes, G.R.   The role of the vestibular system in head-eye coordination. *J. Physiol.*, 246:99-100P, 1975.

3. Gresty, M.A.   Coordination of head and eye movements to fixate continuous and intermittent targets. *Vision Research*, 14:395-403, 1974.

4. Fleming, D.G., Vossius, G.W., Bowman, G., and Johnson, E.L. Adaptive properties of the eye-tracking system as revealed by moving-head and open-loop studies. *Ann. N. Y. Acad. Science*, 156:825-850, 1969.

5. Sugie, N. and Wakakuwa, M.   Visual target tracking with active head rotation. *IEEE Transactions of System Science and Cybernetics*, SSC-6:103-109, 1970.

6. Bizzi, E., Kalil, R.E., Morasso, P., and Tagliasco, V. Central programming and peripheral feedback during eye-head coordination in monkeys. *Bibl. Ophthal.*, 82:220-232, 1972.

7. Morasso, P., Bizzi, E., and Dichgans, J.   Adjustment of saccade characteristics during head movements. *Exp. Brain Res.*, 16: 492-500, 1973.

8. Young, L.R.   Survey of eye movement recording methods. *Behavior Research Methods and Instrumentation*, 7:397-429, 1975.

9. Outerbridge, J.S. and Jones, G M.   Reflex vestibular control of head movement in man. *Aerospace Medicine*, 42:935-940, 1971.

10. Gresty, M.A.   The relationship between head and eye movements. *Agressologie*, 14:7-10, 1973.

11. Bizzi, E., Kalil, R.E., and Morasso, P.   Two modes of active eye-head coordination in monkeys. *Brain Res.*, 40:45-48, 1972.

12. Bizzi, E., Kalil, R.E., and Tagliasco, V.   Eye-head coordination in monkeys: Evidence for centrally patterned organization. *Science*, 173:452-454, 1971.

13. Barr, C.C., Schultheis, L.W., and Robinson, D.A.   Voluntary, non-visual control of the human vestibulo-ocular reflex. *Acta Otolaryngol.*, 81:365-375, 1976.

14. Bizzi, E., Polit, A., and Morasso, P.   Mechanisms underlying achievement of final head position. *J. Neurophysiol.*, 39:435-444, 1976.

15. Bizzi, E. and Schiller, P.H.   Single unit activity in the frontal eye fields of unanesthetized monkeys during eye and head movements. *Exp. Brain Res.*, 10:151-158, 1970.

16. Stryker, M.P. and Schiller, P.H.   Eye and head movements evoked by electrical stimulation of monkey superior colliculus. *Exp. Brain Res.*, 23:103-112, 1975.

17. Robinson, D.A. and Jarvis, D.C.   Superior colliculus neurons studied during head and eye movements of the behaving monkey. *J. Neurophysiol.*, 37:533-540, 1974.

18. Fuller, J.H. and Miles, F.A.   Single unit firing patterns in the vestibular nuclei of alert rhesus monkeys associated with passive whole body rotation, eye movements, and attempted head movements. *Proceedings of the Society for Neuroscience,* p. 217, 1974.

19. Bender, M.B., Shanzer, S., and Wagman, I.H.   On the physiological decussation concerned with head turning. *Confin. Neurol.*, 24:169-181, 1964.

20. Westheimer, G. and Blair, S.M.   Synkinese der augenund kopfbewegungen bei hirnstammreizugen am wachen macacus-affen. *Exp. Brain Res.*, 24:89-95, 1975.

21. Ritchie, L.   The effects of cerebellar lesions on saccadic eye movements. *J. Neurophysiol.*, in press, 1976.

22. Yee, R.D., Zee, D.S., and Cogan, D.G.   Congenital ocular motor apraxia: I. Eye-movement abnormalities. Submitted for publication, 1976.

23. Gresty, M.A.: Eye, head and body movements of the guinea pig in response to optokinetic stimulation and sinusoidal oscillation in yaw. *Pflugers Arch.*, 353:201-214, 1975.

24. Barnes, G. and Benson, A.J.   A model for the prediction of the nystagmus response to angular and linear acceleration stimuli. AGARD-CPP-128 on The Use of Nystagmography in Aviation Medicine, 23:1-13, 1973.

25. Zee, D.S., Optican, L.M., Cook, J., Robinson, D.A., Engel,
     W.K.   Slow saccades in spinocerebellar degeneration. *Arch.
     Neurol.*, 33:243-251, 1976.

26. Vassella, F.,Lutschig, J., and Mumenthaler, M.   Cogan's
     congenital ocular motor apraxia in two successive generations.
     Develop. Med. Child Neurol., 14:788-803, 1972.

27. Atkins, A. and Bender, M.B.   Ocular stabilization during
     oscillatory head movements. *Arch. Neurol.*, 19:559-566, 1968.

28. Dichgans, J., Bizzi, E., Morasso, P., and Tagliasco, V.
     Mechanisms underlying recovery of eye-head coordination
     following bilateral labyrinthectomy in monkeys. *Exp. Brain
     Res.*, 18:548-562, 1973.

29. Dichgans, J., Bizzi, E., Morasso, P., and Tagliasco, V.   The
     role of vestibular and neck afferents during eye-head coordin-
     ation in the monkey. *Brain Res.*, 71:225-232, 1974.

30. J. C.   Living without a balancing mechanism. *New England
     Journal of Medicine*, 246:458-460, 1952.

31. Jongkees, L.B.W.   Cervical vertigo. *Laryngoscope* 79:1473-
     84, 1969.

THE OCULAR MOTOR SYSTEM: NORMAL AND CLINICAL STUDIES

Louis F. Dell'Osso and B. Todd Troost
Department of Neurology, University of Miami
School of Medicine
Miami, Florida

In order to give an appropriate overview of our clinical
studies in the ocular motor system and to exemplify the close
interaction of the clinician and the bioengineer, we will provide
a review of the work of the Miami ocular motor neurophysiology
laboratory, including studies on subjects and patients and the
implications they hold for the control of eye movements.

The framework we will present lends itself to the understanding
of clinical eye signs and conforms to current research findings in
this area. We have aimed at a compromise between the complexities
inherent in these findings and the overly simplified presentations
of most neuro-ophthalmology textbooks. The ocular motor system
consists of two subsystems: version and vergence. The subsystems
give rise to three types of eye movements: fast eye movements
(FEM) and slow eye movements (SEM) from the version subsystem, and
vergence eye movements (VEM) from the vergence subsystem. FEM and
SEM are conjugate whereas VEM are disconjugate. While there are
only these three ocular motor outputs, determined by spatio-
temporal characteristics as well as ocular motorneuronal firing
patterns, there is a multitude of input and pathological stimuli
which may elicit them.

The stimulus usually employed in the laboratory to elicit FEM
is target displacement. The particular FEM which results is
called a voluntary saccade (Dell'Osso and Daroff, 1974). The
latency is approximately 200 milliseconds, and velocity varies
from 30-700 degrees/second and duration from 30 to 100 or more
milliseconds dependent on the amplitude of the saccade, which
normally varies between 0.5 and 40 degrees of visual angle. The

movement is conjugate and ballistic, and the control system is discrete. By that, we mean that even though there is continuous visual information, motor commands are made at some point in time and are by and large irrevocable. The control signal is retinal error. Fig. 1 is a template upon which the various pathways are superimposed, showing FEM as a closed-loop system. With head velocity 0, relative eye position in the head is the same as absolute eye position, and target displacement gives rise to retinal error. A conjugate retinal error sensed by the cortex causes signals to be sent down to the Paramedian Pontine Reticular Formation (PPRF) to initiate the eye movement and reduce the error to 0, in a simple negative feedback system.

Slow eye movements are typically generated in the laboratory during pursuit of a moving target. The resulting SEM is called smooth pursuit (Dell'Osso and Daroff, 1974). Thus, the stimulus is the target motion and the latency between onset of target motion and the movement itself is about 125 milliseconds. The velocity is usually less than 50 degrees/ second. The movement is conjugate and smooth and the control system in this case is continuous, rather than discrete. The control signal is retinal error velocity, sometimes called slip velocity. Referring back to our template (Fig. 1) we have the same interaction of eye position and target position, but a retinal error velocity signal is generated and transmitted to the cortex. A conjugate retinal error velocity again results in signals to the PPRF where a pursuit movement (SEM) is generated.

Another type of SEM (i.e., not smooth pursuit) results from vestibulo-ocular input. The stimulus is head or body motion. The latency is 100 milliseconds or less and velocity may achieve 400 degrees/second. The movement is conjugate and smooth, control is continuous, and is triggered by head acceleration. Fig. 2 is a block diagram which shows the vestibular input summing with the SEM input and FEM velocity commands, and depicts a hypothetical final common integrator. Such an integrator is required for each of these systems, as is the path around the integrator to the ocular motor nuclei and muscle plant. The fast and slow systems are within a feedback loop, but the vestibular system is not. On our template (Fig. 1) head acceleration is shown to cause vestibular input to the brainstem; the resultant output is absolute eye position which is the sum of relative eye position and head position. It is open loop; even though we've indicated the mathematical relationship between head acceleration and head position, this is not a physiological path. If vision is also present, the visual feedback path is closed aroung this loop and the resultant is a combination of open-loop and closed-loop systems operating synergistically.

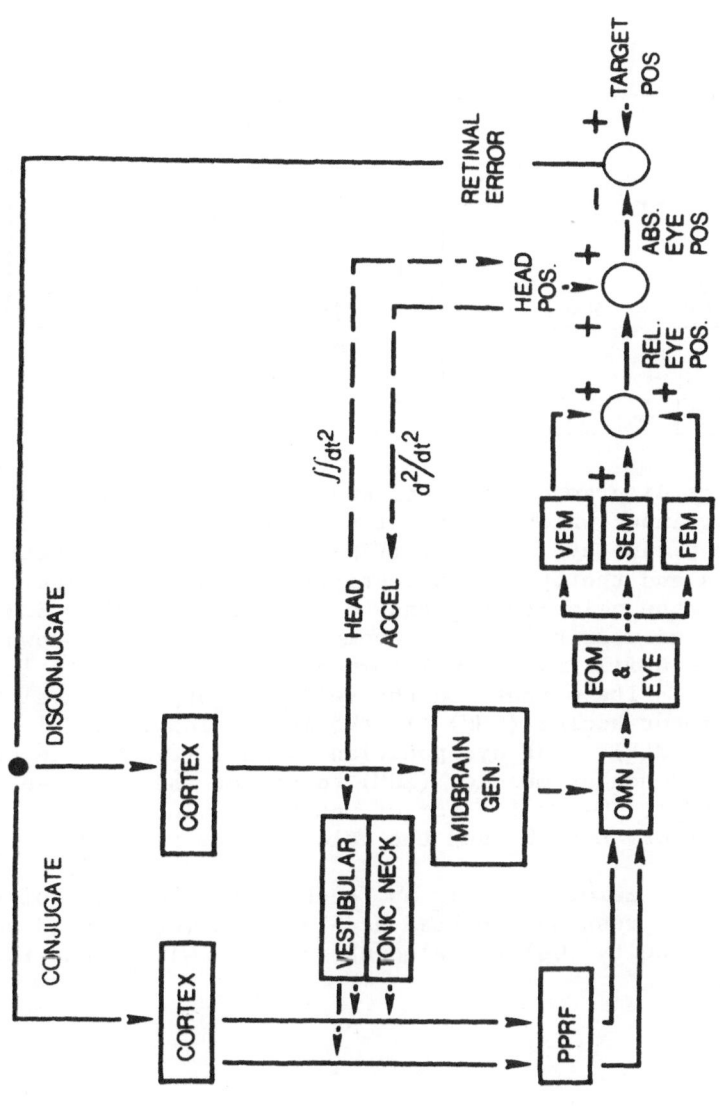

FIGURE 1. Basic block diagram of the ocular motor system with vergence and dual-mode version subsystems. Explanation of the various components are provided in the text.

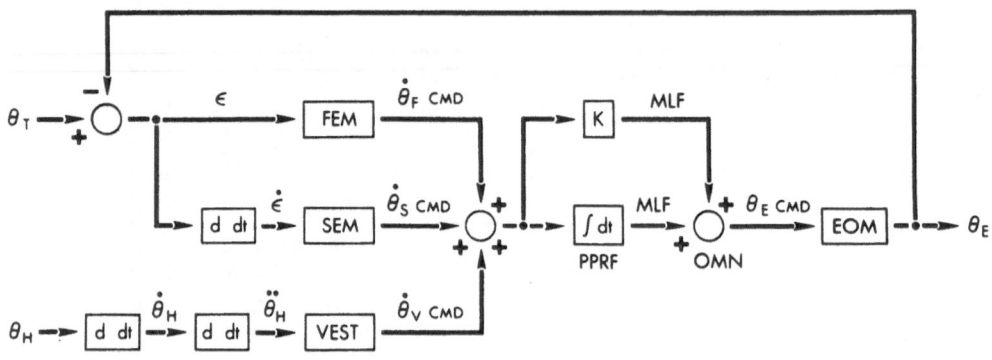

FIGURE 2. Block diagram of the dual-mode version subsystem with
vestibular input which illustrates the difference between the
closed-loop fast eye movement (FEM) and slow eye movement (SEM)
mechanisms and the open-loop vestibulo-ocular apparatus. For
simplicity the velocity commands of the FEM ($\dot{\Theta}_F$ CMD), SEM
($\dot{\Theta}_S$ CMD), and vestibular eye movements ($\dot{\Theta}_V$ CMD) are shown
summing and utilizing a final common integrator ($\int$ dt) located
in the PPRF. Its output and the velocity outputs travel to
the oculomotor nuclei (OMN) via the medial longitudinal
fasciculus (MLF). The eye position command (Θ_E CMD) is sent
to the extra-ocular muscles (EOM) to effect the required eye
position (Θ_E). Θ_T is the target position. In this way, the
position error, $\varepsilon = \Theta_T - \Theta_E$ and the velocity error, $\dot{\varepsilon} = \dfrac{d}{dt}(\Theta_T - \Theta_E)$,

are driven to zero; there is no feedback to the vestibular
system, which responds to head acceleration ($\ddot{\Theta}_H$). Head position
(Θ_H) and velocity ($\dot{\Theta}_H$) are also shown along with their relationship to $\ddot{\Theta}_H$.

The stimuli for vergence eye movements are target displacement or target motion in the Z direction, that is, toward or away from the subject. The latency is 160 milliseconds and the velocity is usually less than 20 degrees/second. The movement is disconjugate but smooth, the control is continuous, and the control signals are either retinal blur or diplopia, or both. Retinal blur is an open-loop input and diplopia is a closed-loop input. On the template (Fig. 1) is the representation of diplopia. A disconjugate retinal error is sensed and gives rise, in the midbrain, to commands to move the eyes disconjugately and thereby reduce the diplopia to 0 by the same negative feedback. In the following material we will look at various clinical abnormalities, and try to relate them to malfunction of the ocular motility control systems.

Referring to Fig. 3, disorders of the FEM subsystem results in signs like opsoclonus, dysmetria, Gegenrücken, macro square wave jerks, and macro saccadic oscillation. Nystagmus (either congenital or acquired) is due to problems of the SEM system, and vestibular malfunction will give rise to vestibular nystagmus. Internuclear ophthalmoplegia (INO) has been discussed previously in this symposium and the implicated lesions in the medial longitudinal fasciculus (MLF) are indicated in Fig. 3.

The earliest studies in our laboratory defined the metric characteristics of horizontal saccadic eye movements in normal adult humans (Weber and Daroff, 1971). Recording from each eye simultaneously, an EOG analysis of horizontal saccades defined their metric characteristics and detailed the trajectory relationships during refixation. Nine distinct left eye - right eye combinations are recognized and analyzed. (Table 1.)

Eye movements that were accurate were defined as normometric, those with errors, as dysmetric. An inverse relationship between amplitude and accuracy emerged as the basic principle of saccadic metrics. Ten degree saccades were normometric in the majority of trials; the remainder primarily represented conjugate under/or overshoot. However, the frequency of normometric saccades decreased significantly at 20 and 30 degrees. As the amplitude increased, conjugate undershooting became more prevalent. Of paramount importance was the finding of disconjugate or disjunctive eye movements, such as involved in a left eye undershoot with simultaneous right eye overshoot. Such observations demonstrate variability and frequently only approximate equality in yoke muscle performance during horizontal saccades. The most common difference in the performance of the two eyes resulted from a monocular error.

Analysis of these errors revealed a distinct tendency toward
adductor overshoot or abductor undershoot. Disconjugate eye
movements occurred in 15% of all trials, although the percentage
in individual subjects varied from 2.0 to 26.2 per cent.

All the dysmetric saccades were followed by a small corrective
movement which accomplished alignment of the fovea with the new
fixation target. Analysis of these correction movements for both
conjugate and disconjugate refixational errors was reported by
Weber and Daroff (1972).

Two types of corrective movements (CM) occurred. One designated
saccadic CM, was fast, had a definite latency, and always followed
conjugate errors. The other was slow, drift-like, without a
latency, and corrected disconjugate refixations. The term glissadic
CM was given to the latter variety.

The saccadic correction was distinctive, easily recognized,
of equal amplitude in both eyes and followed all conjugate errors.
The latencies from the termination of the initial movement until
the onset of the corrective movements were approximately 125 msec.
The latency was similar to saccadic corrections for undershoots
(positive CM) and overshoots (negative CM). The size of the CM
increased monotonically from refixations of 10° to 30°. The glissadic
correction was of low velocity (approximately 20 deg/sec) and
inseparable from the terminal portion of the saccade. There was
therefore no latency between the end of the initial saccade and
the beginning of the correction. Thus two distinct varieties of
CM were defined. These findings suggested certain mechanisms to
explain the corrections accompanying both the conjugate, and in
particular the disconjugate, error. We attempted in our initial
block diagram to explain the different mechanisms that the ocular
motor control system could use to correct disconjugate errors.
Our initial concept of glissades assumed that a disconjugate error
would cause a corrective movement, and it appeared from the records
that these were constant velocity movements rather than the
exponential movements that would reflect the muscle plant. We
were therefore required to explain this phenomenon in the dark as
well as with vision. We could eliminate the visual loop (the
retinal loop) and, since there was no latency, we could also
eliminate the proprioceptive loop (that would require anywhere
from 50-80 milliseconds). The task was reduced to monitoring the
output of the PPRF (the commands to the motor neurons), comparing
this output with the desired eye movement, and when it was decided
that, although the eyes hadn't moved yet, the command was in
error, initiating another command. In this case, disconjugate
saccades would result and the glissade would then appear as a
continuation of the saccade.

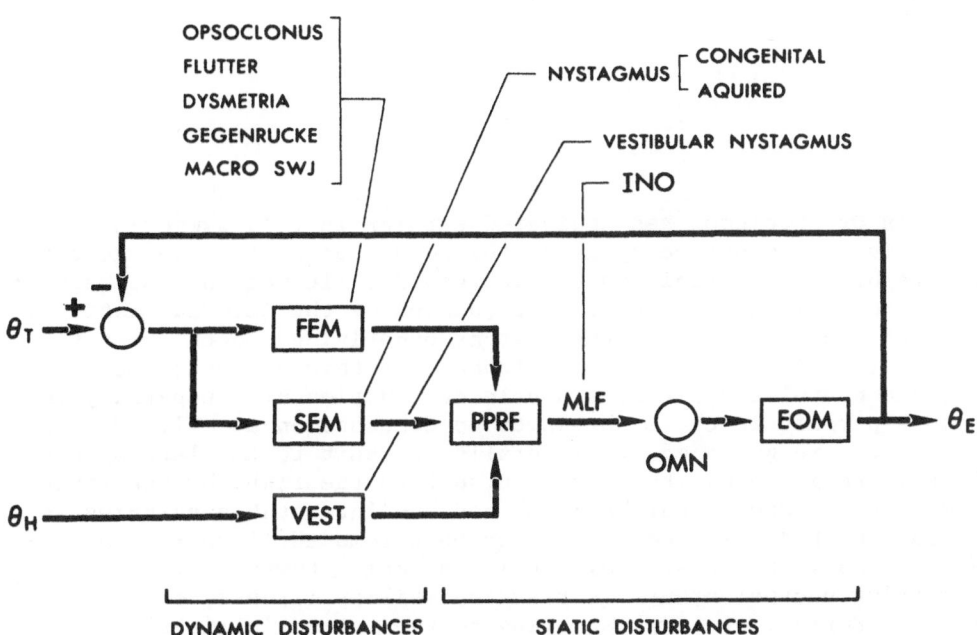

FIGURE 3. Simplified block diagram of the dual-mode version
    subsystem and vestibular input with various ocular motor
    disorders related to disturbances in specific sub-systems.
    Θ_T is target position, Θ_H is head position, and Θ_E is eye
    position.

TABLE 1.   Possible Yoke-pair Combinations

(a) LC-RC   Both eyes correct or "normometric"
(b) LO-RO   Binocular conjugate overshoot
(c) LU-RU   Binocular conjugate undershoot
(d) LU-RC   Left eye undershoot
(e) LC-RU   Right eye undershoot
(f) LO-RC   Left eye overshoot
(g) LC-RO   Right eye overshoot
(h) LU-RO   Left eye under, right eye over
(i) LO-RU   Left eye over, right eye under

As Dr. Robinson has indicated earlier in this symposium, there is some controversy as to the nature of a glissade according to its original definition by old records. It was the analysis of those records that led us to the concept of the internal monitor. A brief consideration of the anatomy underlying smooth pursuit movements will clarify the development of this concept. Earlier notions postulated either a double decussation of the pathway for smooth pursuit in the midbrain or no decussation at all. Pursuit movements are governed ipsilaterally; pursuit to the left by the left posterior hemisphere, and pursuit to the right by the right hemisphere. One of our patients had had intractable seizures as a child, and his left hemisphere had been removed 11 years previously. His refixations appeared clinically normal: however, we noted something unusual about his tracking ability (Troost, et al., 1972). Pursuit of targets moving to the patient's right was smooth, but saccadic or cogwheel pursuit occurred on following to the left. He was unable to match the velocity of targets moving in a leftward direction. We recorded eye movements during pursuit tasks and during refixations to stationary targets. We calculated the gain of his leftward pursuit and found it was low (0.2 - 0.4) despite various target velocities. While tracking sinusoids he similarly showed smooth pursuit to the right but abnormal pursuit to the left (Fig. 4).

Smooth pursuit abnormality is not of localizing value clinically when there is bilateral dysfunction (as often occurs with inattention, diffuse cerebral disease, diffuse brainstem disease or from sedative drugs). However, it is useful in pinpointing a unilateral posterior hemispheric disease to the side of the unindirectional tracking defect. There is usually a contralateral visual field defect as well.

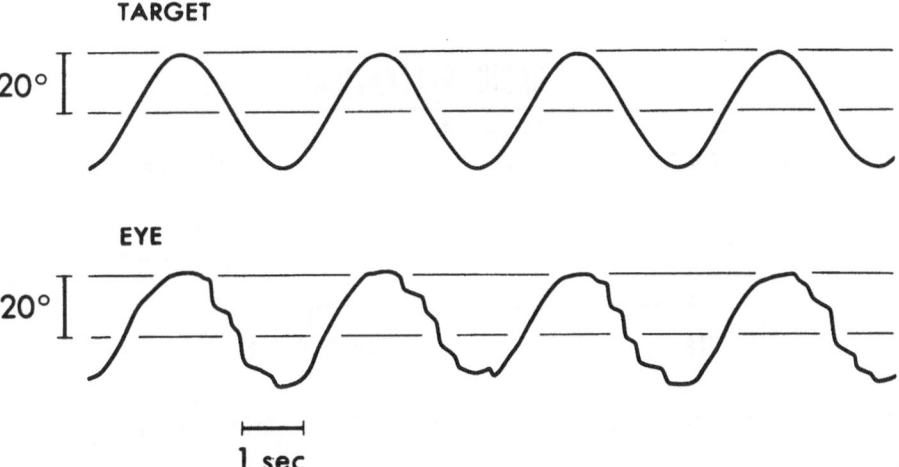

FIGURE 4. Patient with a left hemispherectomy tracking sinusoidally
  moving targets. Pursuit is smooth to the right (up) but
  saccadic or broken to the left (down).

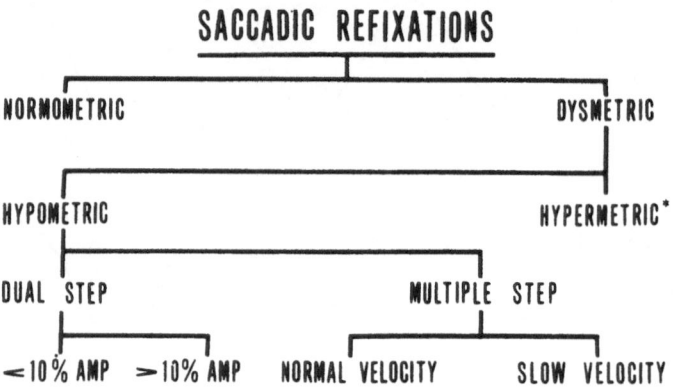

FIGURE 5. Classification of saccadic refixations. *Hypermetric saccades are unusual and have not been completely studied.

Fast eye movements were studied in the patient discussed above (Troost et al., 1972a). The pathway for FEM descends from the hemisphere and crosses in the caudal midbrain or upper pons to the contralateral PPRF. How would an individual with a missing left hemisphere make voluntary saccadic movements? Normally the right hemisphere would produce rapid eye movements in the leftward direction only; however, in this situation the right hemisphere would direct "rehabilitated" saccades in a rightward direction as well. On comparing refixation in rightward and leftward directions the patient made normal leftward saccades, but rightward saccades were abnormal in a number of ways. Accuracy was greatly reduced and only 15% of the eye movements were normometric. A high proportion of them were hypometric, composed of a series of steps, there was a larger number of disjugate errors than is seen in normal subjects, while the velocities of the rightward saccades were within normal limits.

Hypometric saccades themselves were also the subject of analysis (Troost, et al., 1974). Refixations may be classified according to their accuracy and number of corrective movements (Fig. 5). Multiple step hypometric saccades are a common type of hypometric saccade. We consider them pathologic if the velocites of the individual segments are abnormally slow. This variety of hypometric saccade is commonly encountered in patients with diffuse brainstem disease such as Progressive Supranuclear Palsy (PSP). The patient with a left hemispherectomy frequently displayed hypometric saccades during rightward refixations, but the segments had normal velocites and would therefore be considered normal individually. However, since they appeared prominently in 30% of all rightward refixations, their frequency is abnormal.

To review the findings on the hemispherectomy patient, the intact right hemisphere generated the following types of eye movements: 1. Normal rightward pursuit; 2. Defective, low gain, cogwheel pursuit to the left; 3. Normal leftward saccades; 4. Rightward saccades of normal velocity but with great inaccuracy and a high proportion of multiple step hypometric saccades.

A saccadic eye movement has a short period of acceleration, a period of high velocity, and then a short period of deceleration. Examination of activity in the agonist and antagonist muscles reveals that the tonic activity in the agonist goes from a lower level to a higher level, and the antagonist goes from a higher to a lower level. During the saccade a burst of high frequency activity occurs in the agonist which then decays to a tonic level required to hold the eye in a new position, while in the antagonist there is a complete shutoff. It is worthy of note that there is no active breaking. The antagonist does not produce a burst to stop the eye from moving. A requisite to move this highly overdamped

plant in the manner observed is a pulse-step of innervation. If
only a step is applied, a 200 millisecond exponential movement
results. A pulse generator has been postulated which provides a
pulse of information which is then integrated in a neural integrator
pool to get the step. A step is summed with the original pulse,
giving the pulse-step which we see at the ocular motor neurons.
Considering saccadic movements, one notes that they vary in duration
with amplitude; the larger the movement, the longer it takes.
Velocity also increases with amplitude. A study of normal subjects
revealed that the characteristic velocity and amplitude relationship
can be expressed as monotonically increasing and saturating function
(Boghen, et al., 1974). We have calculated two standard deviations
above and below the mean for a large sample of subjects, and our
laboratory regards any eye movements that fall below the lower
border as pathologically slow. There is a great deal of variation
and the variation itself grows with saccadic size. The parameters
of movement are statistically similar for voluntary saccades, fast
phases of optokinetics, fast phases of rotational nystagmus,
vestibular and also caloric-induced nystagmus, and therefore
support our thesis that fast eye movements are a single homogeneous
class (Sharpe et al., 1975). For saccades greater than a few
degrees in amplitude there is a small but statistically significant
difference between saccade velocity in light and dark, and a
similar velocity dependence on structure in the visual field.
Voluntary saccades made in the dark are slower than those made in
the light and the same relation applies for the fast phases of
rotational nystagmus. Summarizing the motor output, the PPRF
sends signals ipsilaterally to the VI nucleus and contralaterally
up the MLF to the III nucleus. Although this view is oversimplified,
it gives the clinician a useful frame of reference when lesions
appear in various locations.

Abnormal eye movements:

     We are primarily concerned here with central supranuclear
defects that cause either a total gaze paralysis (saccades and
pursuit movements absent) or incomplete lesions causing paresis of
gaze. The saccadic or smooth pursuit systems may be affected
separately according to cerebral disease. Saccadic palsy with
normal pursuit occurs in both congenital and acquired ocular motor
apraxia and is presumably due to an abnormality which is bilateral
in the frontomesencephalic projections to the brainstem. Pure
pursuit palsy with entirely normal saccades due to bilateral
posterior hemispheric disease is quite rare. When both fast eye
movements and slow eye movements are paralyzed, it is termed a
gaze palsy.

     A patient with an acquired ocular motor apraxia does not have
rapid eye movements and uses head movements to make refixations

during reading. When required to make refixations during head restraint, the resultant eye movements appear unusually slow. It is unclear clinically whether such eye movements are just very slow saccades, substituted vergence movements or substituted smooth pursuit movements. Vertical eye movements, including saccades, appear frequently entirely intact, at least by crude observation.

Progressive Supranuclear Palsy is a condition characterized by axial rigidity, dementia and a progressive defect in voluntary eye movements. Pathologic examination in the disorder reveals extensive neuronal loss in the basal ganglia, in the paraventricular and periaqueductal regions and in the reticular formation of the brainstem. In some patients there may be paralysis of vertical eye movements (especially in a downward direction) with some preservation of horizontal gaze. We studied a series of such patients (Troost et al., in press), with the following findings: during fixation frequent small to and fro saccades known as square wave jerks or Gegenrücke were present in all patients. The remaining horizontal eye movements were also abnormal, having low velocities and greatly prolonged durations. With head turning the eyes rotate in the opposite direction rather than following with the head as would be the case in an intact subject who was not fixating upon a target. Clinically the refixations often appeared to be hypometric as well as slow. If an observer were not aware whether a saccade or pursuit was being attempted the resultant eye movement would appear the same. The pursuit movements are cogwheel or saccadic and the saccades are hypometric with regular, slow velocity steps. Analysis of eye movement recordings distinguished the two types of output. During a pursuit task there was usually a minimal attempt at following the target. Pursuit was of low gain (0.2 - 0.4) necessitating "catch-up" saccades which were in themselves slow and of long duration; the presence of some definable pursuit made the distinction possible between a tracking attempt and a hypometric saccade. The duration of saccades was greatly prolonged. An eye movement during an attempted 15 degree refixation had a duration of up to 200 msec.

Quantitatively the vestibulo-ocular reflex in these patients was also abnormal. A normal subject can suppress the reflex when he attempts to fixate on a target which rotates with him, but the patient with PSP is unable to do this and has an apparent obligatory compensatory eye movement opposite to the head motion; he is therefore unable to maintain fixation. A normal subject can maintain fixation during head movement by making equal and opposite movements of the eyes within the head. The patient with PSP is unable to maintain fixation; he is not able to make full compensatory eye movements.

Next we will briefly consider some aspects of internuclear ophthalmoplegia (INO). During horizontal refixations the adducting eye either fails to adduct or does so slowly. The abducting eye develops nystagmus with the fast phase in the direction of gaze, with the initial abduction saccade of normal velocity. The slowness of adduction (which may at times be quite subtle) is accentuated during the OKN test. If, for example, the patient has a left INO the left eye will be slow in adduction when the gaze is directed to the right. An optokinetic stimulus passed to the patient's left necessitates repetitive fast eye movements to the right. The right eye (the abducting eye) has normal fast phases but the left (adducting eye) is slow, the difference being readily detectable during the OKN test.

In order to understand optokinetic asymmetry, it is necessary to reconsider how fast phases are generated. We require a pulse and a step of innervation summed together. If only the step occurred without the pulse, the result would be a slow eye movement with exponentially decreasing velocity, reflecting the 200 millisecond plant dynamics. On the other hand, if we had the pulse but not the step, the eye would reach its intended position, would be unable to hold and would drift backwards, resulting in nystagmus. Considering the asymmetry of the abduction and adduction saccades, and superimposing a pursuit movement generated by an optokinetic stimulus moving in the other direction, the result is a clean, brisk, optokinetic response in the abducting eye (Dell'Osso et al., 1974). The adducting eye, still in the process of going to the right (in its fast phase) when the slow phase impinges upon it with a leftward impetus, has a smaller, flat-topped, type of nystagmus. This is the classical Smith and David optokinetic asymmetry sign.

We will now examine the waveforms that accompany congenital nystagmus (CN). We define pendular congenital nystagmus as an ocular motor instability of the slow eye movement subsystem, resulting in periodic motion of the eyes away from and back to the intended gaze angle or target (if there is one), such that the waveform described by the movement is approximately sinusoidal. Occasionally, there are small foveating saccades on the peaks corresponding to target foveation. The object of all nystagmus waveforms is to maximize time-on-target and in that way maximize visual acuity. This strategy on the subject's part must be taken into account when therapy is considered. Our definition of jerk nystagmus similarly involves an ocular motor instability of the slow eye movement subsystem. The result is a periodic drift of the eyes away from the intended gaze angle or target, but a saccade is required in the opposite direction to stop the slow eye movement. We term these breaking saccades. The saccade may either fully refoveate the target, or it may begin another slow eye movement in

the proper direction for refoveation. The direction of jerk
nystagmus is defined as the direction of the corrective saccades
and it is the only waveform parameter that remains constant. All
saccades in nystagmus waveforms are directed toward the target,
and whether or not they achieve foveation is irrelevant. Both the
classical saw-tooth type of jerk nystagmus and pure sinusoidal
nystagmus are very rare in congenital nystagmus, but they are
observed. Fig. 6 shows the three types of pendular nystagmus we
have observed: pure pendular nystagmus, asymmetric pendular
nystagmus (pure pendular sometimes converting to jerk nystagmus)
and pendular with foveating saccades.

    Regarding jerk nystagmus, there are eight types: four
unidirectional and four bidirectional (Dell'Oss and Daroff, 1975).
Of the unidirectional types (Fig. 7), the pure jerk nystagmus
resembles vestibular nystagmus. If, after the foveating saccades,
the eye remains on target for a certain amount of time before its
exponentially increasing velocity drift off target, the result is
a jerk nystagmus with extended foveation. This is conducive to
very good visual acuity. In these two cases, the fast eye movement
brings the eye onto the target. An insufficient amplitude would
only stop the runaway which was taking the eyes away from the
target, and another slow eye movement would return the eye back to
the target again. There would follow a variable period on target
with no motion (good visual acuity) and again, the runaway. Such
a waveform is called pseudocycloid because it resembles a cycloid.
The breaking saccades are of variable amplitude and are occasionally
very small. If they are very small and the slow eye movement
which follows is almost linear, pseudojerk nystagmus results.
Pseudo, not because it is not a jerk nystagmus (it is a jerk
nystagmus since the saccade is directed toward the target), but
because, when examining a patient with this waveform, one invariably
misidentifies its direction. Observation indicates that the fast
phase takes longer than the slow phase and the direction is defined
improperly. In the transition zone between full jerk left and a
full jerk right nystagmus, there are many waveforms that are
variants of bidirectional jerk nystagmus (Fig. 8). They are
almost always called pendular and, without tracings, it is impossible
to tell they are not pendular. Pure pseudopendular nystagmus is
an alternate runaway in each direction, stopped by a breaking
saccade at each end. Thus, there is a slow eye movement runaway
to the right, a breaking saccade to the left, a slow eye movement
runaway to the left, and a breaking saccade to the right. The
target is somewhere in the middle, and very poor visual acuity
accompanies this waveform. In pseudopendular nystagmus with
foveating saccades, the target is at one peak after breaking
saccades which are of variable amplitude; those at the other peaks
are not. These breaking saccades not only stop the runaway but
get the eye on target and there is usually a flat area, indicating

<u>I PENDULAR NYSTAGMUS</u>

A. PURE

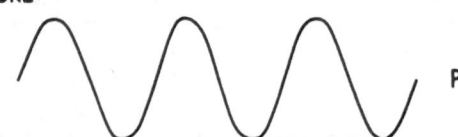

P

B. ASYMMETRIC

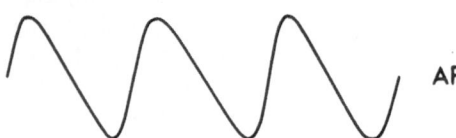

AP

C. WITH FOVEATING SACCADES

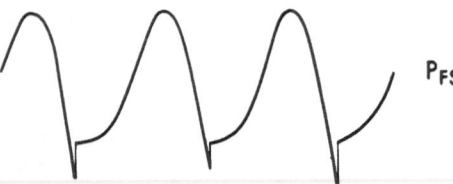

P$_{FS}$

FIGURE 6. The three types of pendular nystagmus: pendular (P),
   asymmetric (AP), and pendular with foveating saccades (PFS).
   Note that although the foveating saccades vary in amplitude
   they all return the eyes to the same point (the target).

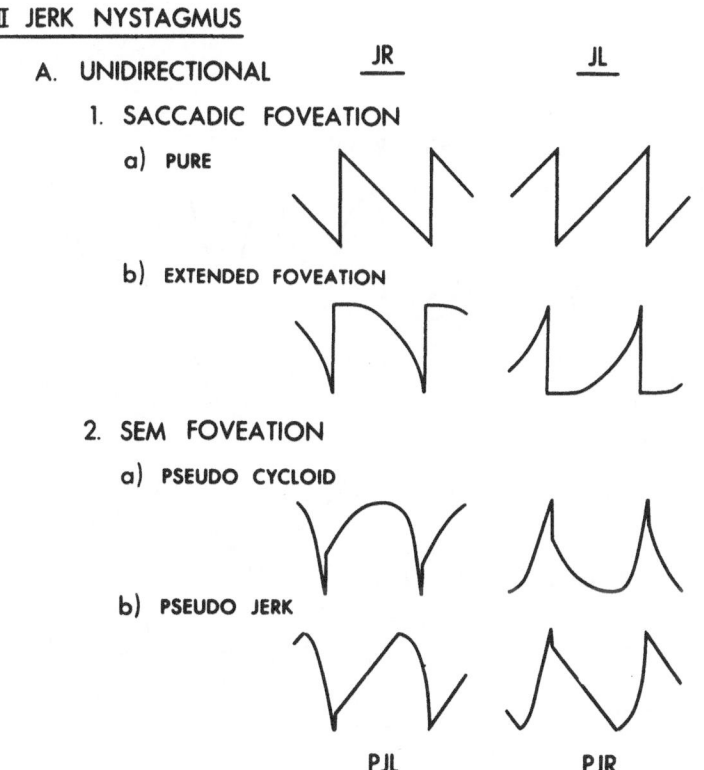

II JERK NYSTAGMUS

   A. UNIDIRECTIONAL   JR   JL

      1. SACCADIC FOVEATION

         a) PURE

         b) EXTENDED FOVEATION

      2. SEM FOVEATION

         a) PSEUDO CYCLOID

         b) PSEUDO JERK

                               PJL   PJR

FIGURE 7. The four unidirectional types of jerk nystagmus: two with saccadic foveation (pure jerk and jerk with extended foveation) and two with slow eye movement foveation (pseudo-cycloid and pseudojerk). Note the reduction in the variability of saccadic amplitude in the pseudocycloid waveform and further reduction in the pueudojerk waveform.

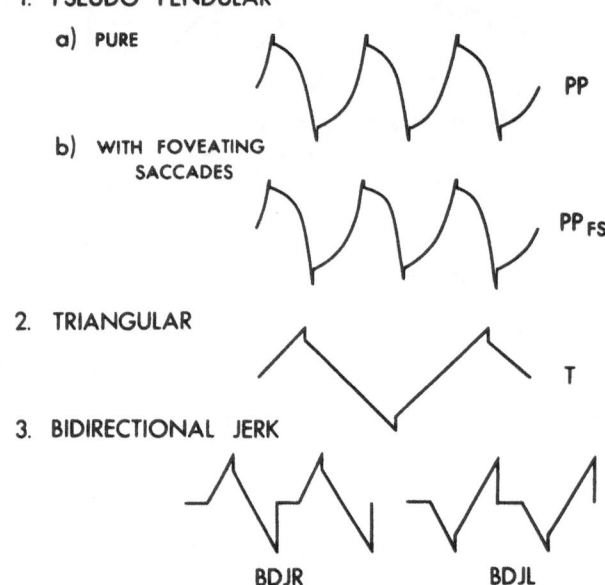

II   JERK NYSTAGMUS

  B.   BIDIRECTIONAL

    1.   PSEUDO PENDULAR

      a) PURE   PP

      b) WITH FOVEATING
          SACCADES   PP FS

    2.   TRIANGULAR   T

    3.   BIDIRECTIONAL JERK

                         BDJR   BDJL

FIGURE 8.   The four types of bidirectional jerk nystagmus: pseudo-
    pendular (PP), pseudopendular with foveating saccades (PPFS),
    triangular (T), and bidirectional jerk (BDJ). All saccades are
    in a corrective direction, i.e., toward the target. The
    foveating saccades of PPFS vary in amplitude but all achieve
    target foveation.

no eye movement, during which the person can see quite well. If
instead of an accelerating runaway, there is a fairly linear
runaway alternating in direction, we have triangular nystagmus;
again with breaking saccades at both ends. Breaking saccades are
always directed towards the target, which is somewhere in the
middle of the waveform which is not good for vision. However,
this form can be sometimes converted to one which is good for
visual acuity. In such a case the saccades are large enough to
achieve the target in one of the directions (assume it's the
rightward direction), and there follows a long period of no eye
movement with good visual acuity. Such a waveform is called
bidirectional jerk right. We have given it a direction although
it is bidirectional, because one of the saccades is a foveating
saccade. Another type involves both pendular and jerk movements.
The jerk nystagmus with pendular oscillation superimposed is
usually a coarse low frequency jerk nystagmus and a fine high
frequency pendular nystagmus superimposed on the slow phase and is
called dual jerk right or dual jerk left (Fig. 9). These two
types of nystagmus, the jerk and the pendular, are relatively
independent. Sometimes convergence will abolish the jerk nystagmus;
the pendular component usually remains although it sometimes also
stops. The relationship of these two components is still under
investigation. Clinically, a patient with CN may manifest a large
zone of apparent pendular nystagmus, which could take any one of
the bidirectional jerk forms, and peripherally show an apparant
jerk nystagmus which may or may not be real. If he has such a
large "pendular" neutral zone, the clinician is tempted to identify
a case of pendular nystagmus. If on the other hand he has a very
narrow neutral zone, the diagnosis may be jerk nystagmus; he may
have jerk in lateral gaze and have one of the pseudopendular
waveforms, which will be diagnosed as pendular, in the middle gaze
positions. In the absence of eye movement recordings, the tendency
therefore is to over-diagnose pendular nystagmus and under-
diagnose jerk nystagmus. Consequently many speculative correlations
between sensory defects and nystagmus must be re-evaluated in the
light of objective criteria in the form of accurate eye movement
recordings. On this basis, we have concluded that all nystagmus
is a motor defect, no matter what the waveform is.

     Macro square wave jerks are exemplified by a woman with
demyelinating disease who has bilateral INO (Dell'Osso et al.,
1975). On examination of the eye movement recordings (Fig. 10),
we see that there is spurious saccade to the left, followed by a
return saccade to the right after a very short latency (80 milliseconds). The subject remains on target for a period of time
before another saccade is initiated. These are macro square wave
jerks; the fact that they are not very square is because the INO
is bilateral. It is evident that the abducting saccades have
higher velocity peaks than the adducting saccades, both eyes

abducting faster than they adduct. This instability belongs to the
fast system, such that there is a spurious saccade away from the
target (in this case off to the left), followed by a rapid corrective
saccade to the right and finally a longer period of time on the
target. After we discovered that the macro square wave jerks
occurred in the dark, we knew it wasn't retinal information that
was generating the corrective saccade. Nor could we depend on
feedback from eye position because the conjugate return saccade
would have to be programmed according to information based on
asymmetric eye positions due to the INO. We were led to the model
shown in Fig. 11. We postulated that the disturbance in the right
PPRF pulse generator (the solid lines trace the activity) would
generate the saccadic movement to the left in both eyes. This is
sensed by an internal monitor that monitors the position command
going to the ocular motor nuclei and compared it to the desired
position of the eyes (based on retinal information). After the
spurious saccade, an error is detected, sent across the other side
to the pulse generator and, with very short latency, the corrective
saccade (in the dashed lines) returns the eyes to target. This is
an example of the application of simple models to the understanding
of pathological eye movements.

III DUAL JERK NYSTAGMUS

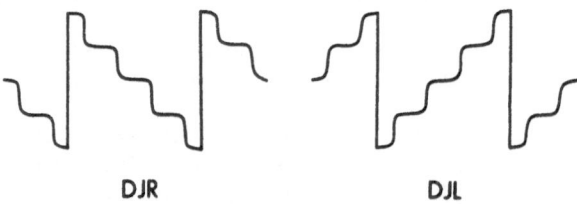

DJR   DJL

FIGURE 9. Dual jerk nystagmus showing sinusoidal modulation of
    the slow eye movement off target.

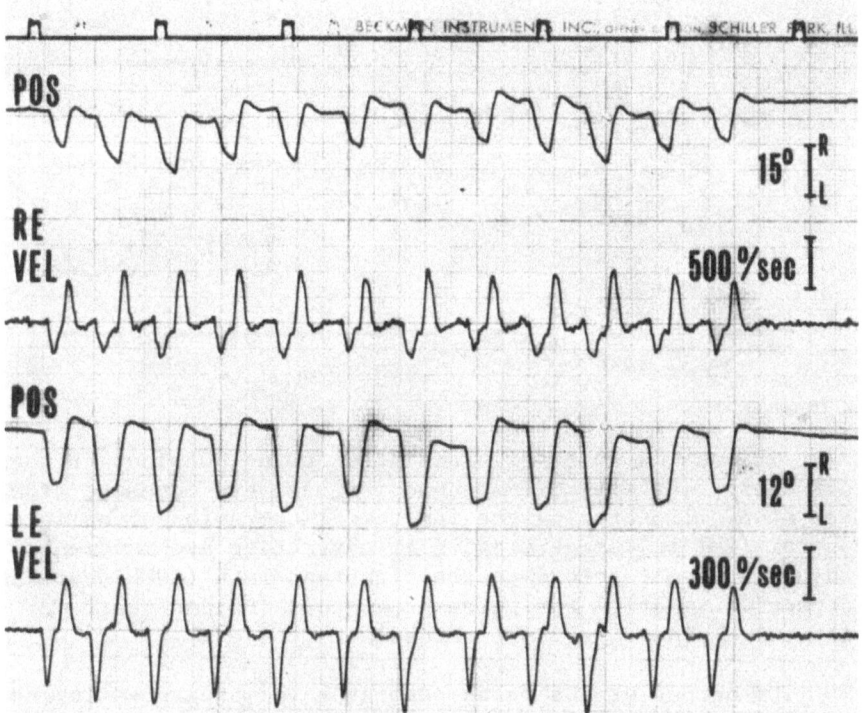

FIGURE 10. Binocular position (POS) and velocity (VEL) recordings
    of macro square wave jerks showing their unidirectional nature
    relative to the intended gaze position evident at the beginning
    and end of the POS traces. The oscillation consists of a
    leftward saccade that moves the eyes off the target and is
    followed, after a variable but brief latency, by a corrective
    rightward saccade which results in refoveation. The patient's
    bilateral internuclear ophthalmoparesis, with the right eye
    (RE) more affected than the left (LE), is apparent in both the
    POS and VEL waveforms. Different calibration for the two eyes
    should be noted and is explained in the text. The timing
    marks at the top indicate 1 second intervals.

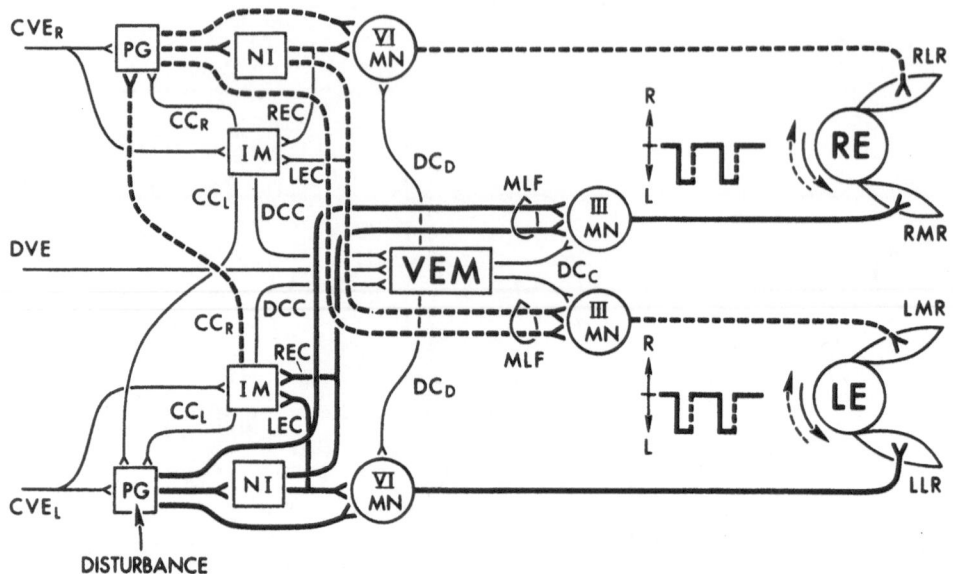

FIGURE 11. Binocular model of brain-stem output portions of the
   horizontal fast eye movement and vergence eye movement (VEM)
   subsystems illustrating the functional operation of an internal
   monitor (IM) in the generation of corrective eye movements.
   Conjugate visual errors to the right and left (CVER and CVEL,
   respectively) drive the pulse generators (PG) on their
   respective side to produce saccades.

     The output of the pulse generator is integrated in the
neural integrator (NI) and the resulting step of innervation
is summed with the original pulse from the pulse generator at
the motoneuron (MN). (Motoneuronal summing is provided for
simplicity only; summing may actually occur at a prenuclear
level.) Signals then go to the respective extraocular muscles
(RLR, RMR, LMR, LLR) to drive the right (RE) and the left (LE)
eyes. Disconjugate visual errors (DVE) drive the vergence eye
movement subsystem to produce disconjugate commands of convergence (DCC) and divergence (DCD). The IM monitors the
commands to both eyes (REC and LEC), compares them with the
desired output (CVE), and directs the required conjugate
correction to the right (CCR) or left (CCL) pulse generator
as well as any required disconjugate corrective command (DCC)
to the vergence eye movement subsystem. The disturbance
input for this patient and the pathways for the consequent
abnormal leftward saccade are in heavy solid lines, with the
pathways for the corrective rightward saccade in dashed lines.
The resulting macro square wave jerks are shown next to each
eye. For simplicity, we have not diagrammed the internuclear
ophthalmoparesis.

REFERENCES

Boghen, D., Troost, B.T., Daroff, R.B., Dell'Osso, L.F. and
    Birkett, J.E. Velocity characteristics of normal human
    saccades. *Invest. Ophthal.*, 13:619-623, 1974.

Dell'Osso, L.F., and Daroff, R.B. Congenital nystagmus waveforms
    and foveation strategy. *Doc. Ophthal.*, 39:155-182, 1975.

Dell'Osso, L.F., and Daroff, R.B. Functional organization of the
    ocular motor system. *Aerospace Med.*, 45:873-875, 1974.

Dell'Osso, L.F., Robinson, D.A., and Daroff, R.B. Optokinetic
    asymmetry and internuclear ophthalmoplegia. *Arch. Neurol.*,
    31:138-139, 1974.

Dell'Osso, L.F., Troost, B.T., and Daroff, R.B. Macro square
    wave jerks. *Neurol.*, 25:975-979, 1975.

Sharpe, J.E., Troost, B.T., Dell'Osso, L.F., and Daroff, R.B.
    Comparative velocities of different types of fast eye movements
    in man. *Invest. Ophthal.*, 14:689-692, 1975.

Troost, B.T., Daroff, R.B., and Dell'Osso, L.F. Quantitative
    analysis of the ocular motor deficit in progressive supranuclear
    palsy (PSP). In press, *Trans. Am. Med. Assoc.*

Troost, B.T., Daroff, R.B., Weber, R.B., and Dell'Osso, L.F.
    Hemispheric control of eye movements. II. Quantitative
    analysis of smooth pursuit in a hemispherectomy patient.
    Arch. Neurol., 27:449-452, 1972.

Troost, B.T., Weber, R.B., and Daroff, R.B. Hemispheric control
    of eye movement. I. Quantitative analysis of refixation
    saccades in a hemispherectomy patient. *Arch. Neurol.*, 27:
    441-448, 1972a.

Troost, B.T., Weber, R.B., and Daroff, R.B. Hypometric saccades.
    Amer. J. Ophthal., 78:1002-1005, 1974.

Weber, R.B., and Daroff, R.B. Corrective movements following
    refixation saccades: type and control system analysis.
    Vision Res., 12:467-475, 1972.

Weber, R.B., and Daroff, R.B. The metrics of horizontal saccadic
    eye movements in normal humans. *Vision Res.*, 11:921-928,
    1971.

IS THE CEREBELLUM TOO OLD TO LEARN?

D. A. Robinson
The Wilmer Institute
Department of Ophthalmology
The Johns Hopkins School of Medicine
Baltimore, Maryland

When people get a new prescription for glasses that involves a sudden increase of several diopters, they often complain of dizziness and disorientation. Fortunately, it disappears in a few days. What caused it? Well, suppose the new glasses magnified everything by 20%. If the patient turns his head to the left at 100 deg/sec (a modest velocity) the visual world turns to the right (relative to the head) at 120 deg/sec, with his new glasses on. But the vestibuloocular reflex (vor) is only moving the eyes in a compensatory movement at 100 deg/sec to the right, just like it used to before the new glasses. Thus, the images of the world now appear to slip to the right at 20 deg/sec.

The illusion that the visual world is not stationary is not funny. It is nauseating. It is the key element in motion sickness. Clinically, it is called oscillopsia. It takes years for some patients with acquired involuntary eye movements (e.g. downbeat nystagmus) to get used to the idea that the world is not really moving. So the person with a sudden 20% magnification feels nauseous because his new glasses give him oscillopsia. The fact that this discomfort disappears in a few days is interesting. How does that happen?

Melvill Jones (Gonshor and Melvill Jones, 1976) and his colleagues investigated this problem. He heard about psychologists who wore reversing prisms! These Dove prisms reverse the seen world from left to right so if the head goes at 100 deg/sec to the left, the seen world also goes at 100 deg/sec to the left, not the right as happens normally. If the vor makes normal "compensatory" movements the retinal slip is 200 deg/sec. That's oscillopsia!

Yet these psychologists went mountain climbing while wearing reversing prisms! How could they do that with such gross oscillopsia? Melvill Jones et al. studied the vor of such subjects. They found that the brain would not put up for long with such nonsense. It rewired the vor backwards so the eyes move in the "wrong" direction but now, at least, they move in the direction that lessens retinal slip and so improves clear vision during head movements.

This incredible plasticity of a "simple three neuron arc" astounded many vestibular physiologists but it has now been proven again and again that the vor is plastic (e.g. Miles and Fuller, 1974; Gauthier and Robinson, 1975) in rabbit, cat, monkey and man. This plasticity is measured by determining the gain g of the vor which is eye velocity divided by head velocity. If the reflex is working normally then g is 1.0. Prisms and lenses disrupt eye-head coordination because the eye no longer goes at the velocity that is needed to hold images still on the retina. This is a form, if you like, of artificially induced vestibuloocular dysmetria. It causes oscillopsia. The brain reacts by changing g until images no longer slip around on the retina during head movements and oscillopsia ceases. For example, if 2X telescope lenses are put on an animal, images move twice as fast on the retina as normal. To stop this, g must increase from 1.0 to 2.0. And that's what happens. If reversing prisms are worn then g must reverse and go to -1.0 to stop images from slipping. And that's nearly what happens. The process takes roughly eight days.

The result of all this is to reveal a plastic control mechanism in the brain that, on the basis of experience (oscillopsia) learns to adapt the vor to the new conditions. Of course, it is not "learning" in the sense in which psychologists use the term. Technically, it is a parametric adaptive control system but the term motor learning is useful to emphasize that motor behavior is shaped by sensory experience. Naturally, this system did not evolve to deal with lenses and prisms but to deal with vestibulo-ocular dysmetria resulting from natural causes that 80 odd years of wear and tear on the nervous system create (e.g., cell attrition from trauma and diseases). The operation of this repair process is seen particularly clearly in the vor because this reflex is open loop. There aren't a lot of local and suprasegmental feedback loops as there are in spinal motor control systems which act as fast error correcting devices. There is only a feedforward path from the canals to the eye muscles. There isn't even any local stretch receptor feedback from the muscles. Thus, as Ito (1972) pointed out, the existence of a mechanism to maintain the proper gain of this reflex could be hypothesized on purely theoretical grounds.

Ito further proposed a mechanism for this control. The canal signal projects to the vestibulocerebellum on mossy fibers (mf) as shown in Fig. 1 and causes Purkinje cells to modulate in lock-step with the canal signal. They, in turn, inhibit cells in the vestibular nucleus (vn). If the depth of modulation of Purkinje cells changes, then the gain of the whole reflex would change (β path, Fig. 1). This offers a nice mechanism for changing the gain of the vestibuloocular reflex and, for example, Lisberger and Fuchs (1974) have shown that monkeys evidently use it for visual suppression of the vor. But here we are concerned not with rapid on-line modulation of the reflex but slow, long-term, semipermanent changes in the gain.

However, this mechanism would be useless if it did not know when to change the gain and by how much. The error (oscillopsia) created by dysmetria (wrong gain) is, of course, detected by the visual system which (Fig. 1) compares the position of gaze, G, to the position of objects in the seen world, W. Movement of the retinal images excites directionally selective cells whose discharge rate reflects retinal slip velocity, ė. Ito reasoned that retinal slip must project to the vestibulocerebellum if that signal is to be used to readjust the gain. Maekawa and Simpson (1973), in Ito's laboratory, looked for and found just such a projection; it runs on ganglion cell axons (in the rabbit) down the accessory optic tract (aot, Fig. 1) to terminate in the nucleus of the optic tract (not; Hoffmann et al., 1976). From there it projects to the inferior olive (io) and is relayed to the vestibulocerebellum on climbing fibers (cf).

Thus, all of the pieces were in place for this scheme but one now had to make an important additional assumption. Obviously, if plastic changes occur, there must be modifiable synapses somewhere in the vor. This scheme puts those synapses in the cerebellum between the parallel T fibers and the Purkinje cells. This is a key part of the hypothesis because if it's true it will have important and far-reaching consequences for cerebellar physiology not only in eye movement control but in motor control in general.

I set out to do a very simple and obvious test of this theory (Robinson, 1976). I put reversing prisms on cats. They wore these goggles all day every day while walking around the laboratory and for 2 hours each day, they were restrained in a box and forcibly rotated en bloc, sinusoidally at 0.05 Hz with a peak head velocity of 30 deg/sec. In about eight days the gain of the vor fell from 0.9 to 0.1 and stabilized. The gain did not reverse and this may be due to plastic changes in optokinetic responses and the use of neck proprioception in stabilizing vision during self-generated head movements. My only concern was to make a large, unequivocal

change in gain. When the flocculus and nodulus were removed the
gain rose to about 1.1 and when the whole prism-wearing experiment
was repeated, there was no change in gain at all.

So this supported the theory by at least showing that the
vestibulo-cerebellum is necessary for this plastic-adaptive behavior
to occur. In other experiments, it appeared that of the two, the
nodulus was more important than the flocculus. In fact, in the
cat, if only the flocculi are removed, plasticity is fully retained.
However, it does not prove, only suggests, that the seat of the
plasticity is in the vestibulocerebellum.

The question of whether modifiable synapses are in the cerebellum remains unresolved at this time. The situation became confused
recently by results on a different type of vestibuloocular repair
process. When the vestibular nerve is sectioned, the vertigo,
nystagmus and generalized postural and motor disturbances which
occur are compensated in a few days to a few weeks depending on
species and age. The nystagmus is also a form of vestibuloocular
dysmetria and compensation is another form of plastic adaptation.
It seemed to me that this type of adaptation had several advantages
over gain control. It was more natural since the animal was
recovering from a real lesion, not dysmetria artificially induced
by lenses and prisms. It also avoided the tedious process of
prism adaptation. So, it seemed that it might have been easier to
pursue the quest for the modifiable synapse in the vestibulocerebellum with such a paradigm.

But first, it was necessary to find out whether the vestibulocerebellum had anything to do with the repair of VIIIth nerve
lesions. A review of the literature left one unsure. Several
reports indicated that compensation still took place without the
cerebellum but those studies usually were not quantitative and it
was possible that the time course of recovery could be quite
different with and without the cerebellum. However, a recent
report by Schaefer and Meyer (1974) made even this unlikely. They
found that after a lesion nystagmus in the guinea pig disappeared
almost as rapidly after the cerebellum was removed as before.
Nevertheless, G. Haddad and I decided to check this out in the cat
in which, with our accurate method of measuring eye movements, we
could follow the time course of slow phase eye velocity. And, of
course, we removed only the vestibulocerebellum (mainly the
flocculus and nodulus).

I'm afraid we confirmed our fears. We made electrolytic, and
so partial, lesions in chronically prepared alert cats. Normal
cats recovered from VIIIth nerve lesions in about three days and
cats without a vestibulocerebellum recovered in approximately the
same amount of time. There was an indication that recovery was
slightly slower and less complete in the latter case. A manuscript

which will describe all this more exactly is in preparation but the upshot of it all is that the vestibulocerebellum has little or nothing to do with the recovery from VIIIth nerve lesions.

As a double check, Haddad showed that the same vestibulocerebellectomized cat that had recovered from an VIIIth nerve lesion, showed no plasticity in the gain of its vor when tested with reversing prisms. From this we can safely conclude that, in the cat, the mechanism that effects plastic changes in gain requires an intact vestibulocerebellum, the mechanism that rebalances the vestibular system after an VIIIth nerve lesion does not.

Llinás et al. (1975) performed a more extensive series of experiments on the recovery of VIIIth nerve lesions in the rat. Their major finding was that recovery depended on the integrity of the inferior olive and deep cerebellar nuclei but not on the cerebellar cortex. The necessity of the climbing fiber system, of course, fits in nicely with the theory in Fig. 1 but the fact that cerebellar cortex (e.g., the vestibulocerebellum) is not needed indicates again that there is a basic difference between gain repair and VIIIth nerve lesion repair.

This means that we are no closer to an answer to the question about modifiable synapses in the cerebellum and, for the present, all we can do is speculate. Returning to gain control and Fig. 1, there are three fairly obvious alternatives to putting modifiable synapses in the cerebellum. The learning process (modifiable synapses) could be located somewhere else in the brain. That circuit would prepare the necessary signal which must be added to or subtracted from the presumed inaccurate canal signal to produce the correct eye velocity command. That correction signal must go through the vestibulocerebellum so it must arrive there on either climbing fibers or mossy fibers. One possibility, the climbing fibers, can probably be ruled out on the grounds that they fire too slowly. To double the vor gain, for example, one must add a peak modulation of about 50 spikes/sec to Purkinje cell firing rates during one half cycle (of sinusoidal head rotation) and decrease it by the same amount on the other half cycle. Since there is, in general, only one climbing fiber for each Purkinje cell, it is simply impossible for the former, firing at 1-4 spikes/ sec to induce a 100 spike/sec modulation in the rate of the latter.

Another peculiarity of climbing fibers that makes it unlikely that they carry high speed, deep modulation signals is that each climbing fiber climbs everywhere over the entire dendritic tree of a single Purkinje cell. This blanketing of one cell by another is unique in neuron cytoarchitecture. If all the climbing fiber wanted to do was fire the Purkinje cell with a synaptic security of one, this arborization is ridiculous overkill. All one needs

is several large synapses near the axon hillock or initial segment.
The fact that a climbing fiber goes everywhere that parallel T
fibers synapse on a Purkinje cell makes one suspect that the
climbing fiber has some business with those synapses, not the
Purkinje cell itself.

A second possibility is to suppose that the learned behavior
arrived on climbing fibers not as a correction signal but in a
more subtle form such as a change from, say, 1-2 spikes/sec to 3-4
spikes/sec. But this change in steady level could only change the
gain of the vor if it changed the synaptic strengths of the
parallel T fibers. Thus, we would have modifiable synapses in the
cerebellum but they may not be plastic. The plasticity could
still be central to the inferior olive. But, of course, the gain
changes of the modifiable synapses must outlast the individual
climbing fiber spikes and respond to their time average. Since
the mechanism of gain change probably would have to involve bio-
chemical changes in, say, properties of the subsynaptic membranes,
one might expect the gain changes to respond quite slowly to
climbing fiber activity so that if the latter suddenly stopped
firing, the change may persist for a few seconds to a few minutes.
If it persisted for a few days, then we would say that plasticity
resided in the cerebellum. If it persisted for a few hours, one
gets into a gray area where it becomes necessary to define
plasticity more carefully. The point here is that modifiable
synapses and plastic modifiable synapses are conceptually quite
different and one must be prepared in future tests to distinguish
between short-term and semi-permanent modifiability.

Finally, there is the possibility that the correction signal
arrives on mossy fibers. The problem with this is that the correction signal must be a good copy of the head velocity signal (from
the canals). Since that signal already projects directly to the
vestibulocerebellum, it seems a bit odd to send it somewhere else,
operate on it plastically and return it to the cerebellum. However,
other theories of how vision interacts with the vestibuloocular
reflex, do in fact lead to circuits with such a potential.

In Fig. 1, the eye velocity command $\dot{E}'$, is proposed to project,
as an efferent copy signal, to a system (vvi) in which retinal
slip velocity $\dot{e}$ is also used to judge the relative motion of seen
objects. For example, if $\dot{E}'$ and $\dot{e}$ are simply added, the result is
the motion of a seen object with respect to the head. Now assume
this signal projects to the vestibulocerebellum on mossy fibers.
This now allows vision (Lisberger and Fuchs, 1974) or even the
attempt to visually localize in the dark (Barr et al., 1976) to
modulate Purkinje cell activity and alter eye velocity.

Specifically, during normal use of the vor, $\dot{E}'$ and $\dot{H}'$ are
signals equal but opposite in sign. If they projected through

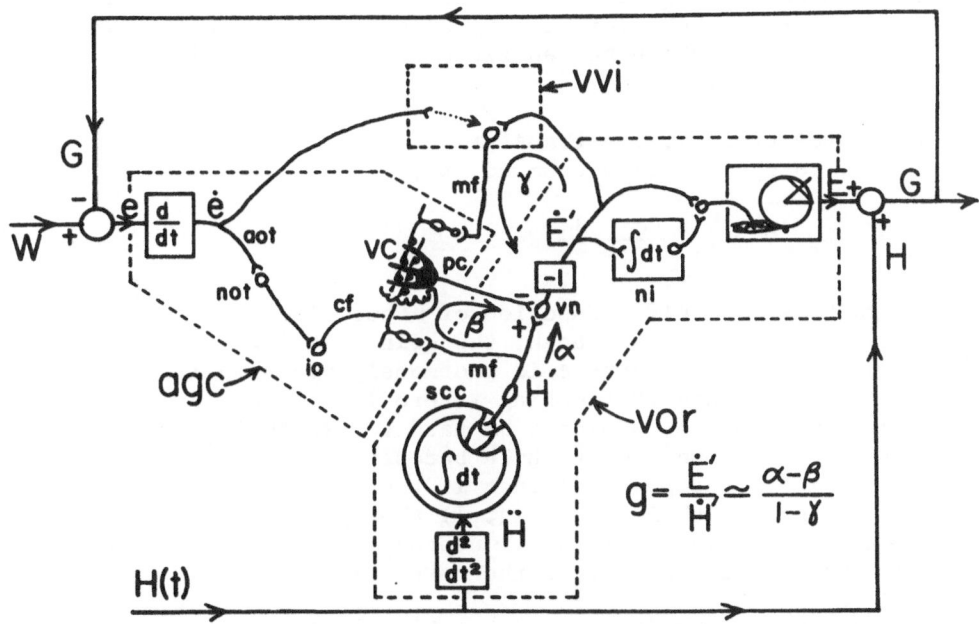

FIGURE 1. The vestibuloocular reflex (vor) is kept in proper
operation by an automatic gain control circuit (agc) which
may also be modulated by another form of visual–vestibular
interaction (vvi). The semicircular canals respond to head
acceleration, Ḧ, integrate it and send a head velocity signal
Ḣ' into the vestibular nucleus (vn) with gain α . When its
sign is changed (-1) this signal constitutes an eye velocity
command Ė'. This is integrated again by a neural integrator
(ni) and produces a change in eye position, E, that is equal
and opposite to head position, H, so that the gaze axis, G,
remains stable in space.

It's proposed that agc starts at the retina where the
position of objects in the seen world W are compared to G and
the rate of change or retinal slip, ė, is extracted and sent
through the nucleus of the optic tract (not) via the accessory
optic tract (aot) to the inferior olive (io) and to the
vestibulocerebellum (vc) and climbing fibers (cf). Head
velocity Ḣ' is also sent to vc on mossy fibers (mf). The gain
of this loop through Purkinje cells (pc) is β. It is proposed
that an efference copy of Ė' is sent to vvi and relayed back
to vc on mossy fibers with gain γ.

paths β and γ to the Purkinje cells, their effects would cancel out, Purkinje cells would modulate little and would not alter the gain of the basic vor. But, if vision or perception could turn off the γ path, then the β path would be unopposed, the Purkinje cell would modulate vigorously and cancel or suppress the vor. This is the sort of behavior seen by Miles, when recording from Purkinje cells, and which he describes elsewhere in this conference proceedings.

More analytically, the transfer function from the canal output, $\dot{H}'$, to eye velocity command, $\dot{E}'$, is

$$g \simeq \frac{\dot{E}'}{\dot{H}'} = \frac{\alpha - \beta}{1 - \gamma}$$

so that gain is not only a function of β but also of γ . If β increases or γ decreases or both, the gain goes down and vice versa. Obviously, this scheme is enormously oversimplified. The reader can see at once that making γ zero is not sufficient to make the gain zero. It wouldn't be hard to fix that up with more assumptions but it isn't worthwhile because all this is already too speculative. The point is that if there were modifiable synapses in the γ path in vvi (Fig. 1) then gain control could still take place which would still depend on the cerebellum but plastic synapses need not be in the cerebellum.

At this point the story ends. I have explored some of the obvious alternative explanations. The idea that motor learning takes place through modifiable synapses so that the cerebellum can repair dysmetria is an attractive idea clinically since it emphasizes the role of the cerebellum, not in creating movements but in coordinating them and modulating them to make them orthometric. Obviously, motor learning need be only one of many functions of the cerebellum.

Whether or not the modifiable synapses are in the cerebellum, the experiments described here indicate that cerebellar pathways are needed for the repair of some types of dysmetria. This focuses attention on repair itself and the fact that when one sees, clinically, dysmetria that is not repaired (persisting signs of incoordination of slow onset) it suggests that the lesion is either distal to the available repair mechanism (e.g., a VIth nerve palsy or internuclear ophthalmoplegia) or the lesion has become so large that the repair circuits can no longer keep up (e.g., large pontine lesions) or cerebellar circuits themselves are involved so that malfunctioning circuits can no longer be repaired (saccadic dysmetria from cerebellar lesions might be an example of this). This adds an interesting but complicating aspect to the interpretation of oculomotor disorders of cerebellar origin.

REFERENCES

Barr, C.C., Schultheis, L.W. and Robinson, D.A. Voluntary, non-
    visual control of the human vestibuloocular reflex. *Acta
    Otolaryngologica,* 81:365-375, 1976.

Gauthier, G.M. and Robinson, D.A. Adaptation of the human vestibulo-
    ocular reflex to magnifying lenses. *Brain Res.,* 92:331-335,
    1975.

Gonshor, A. and Melvill Jones, G. Extreme vestibuloocular
    adaptation induced by prolonged optical reversal of vision.
    J. Physiol., 256:381-414, 1976.

Hoffmann, K.P. Behreud, K. and Schoppmann, A. A direct afferent
    visual pathway from the nucleus of the optic tract to the
    inferior olive in the cat. *Brain Res.,* 115:150-153, 1976.

Ito, M. Neural design of the cerebellar motor control system.
    Brain Res., 40:81-84, 1972.

Lisberger, S.G. and Fuchs, A.F. Response of flocculus Purkinje
    cells to adequate vestibular stimulation in alert monkey;
    fixation vs. compensatory eye movements. *Brain Res.,* 69:347-
    353, 1974.

Llinás, R., Walton, K., Hillman, D.E. and Sotelo, C.   Inferior
    olive: its role in motor learning. *Science,* 190:1230-1231,
    1975.

Maekawa, K. and Simpson, J.I. Climbing fiber responses evoked
    in vestibulocerebellum of rabbit from visual system. *J.
    Neurophysiol.,* 36:649-666, 1973.

Miles, F.A. and Fuller, J.H. Adaptive plasticity in the vestibulo-
    ocular responses of the rhesus monkey. *Brain Res.,* 80:512-
    516, 1974.

Robinson, D.A. Adaptive gain control of vestibuloocular reflex
    by the cerebellum. *J. Neurophysiol.,* 39:954-969, 1976.

Schaefer, K.P. and Meyer, D.L. Compensation of vestibular lesions,
    In *Handbook of Sensory Physiol.,* vol. VI/2: *Vestibular
    System.* Part 2: *Psychophysics, Applied Aspects and General
    Interpretations.* H.H. Kornhuber (editor), Springer-Verlag,
    page 463-490, 1974.

THE PRIMATE FLOCCULUS AND EYE-HEAD COORDINATION

F. A. Miles
Laboratory of Neurophysiology
National Institute of Mental Health
Bethesda, Maryland   20014

As a part of the classical vestibular cerebellum receiving a direct projection from the semicircular canals, the flocculus has long been thought to be implicated in the vestibular stabilization of the eyes. Anatomical and physiological studies in the cat and rabbit have generated a wealth of information about its relationship with brainstem vestibuloocular pathways, and there is currently considerable interest in the flocculus as the probable site of modifiable elements concerned with the long-term maintenance of appropriate vestibuloocular reflexes. Recent electrophysiological studies in the awake monkey, however, seem to indicate that the flocculus is also involved in other, previously unsuspected, aspects of oculomotor function. Before reviewing these new developments, I shall briefly describe the basic neuronal circuitry involved. For more extensive treatments of the latter, the reader is referred to a number of excellent review articles (1,2,3).

FLOCCULO-VESTIBULO-OCULAR CIRCUITRY

In recent years, the flocculus has come to be regarded as an inhibitory side-loop of the horizontal vestibuloocular pathway, receiving a mossy fibre primary vestibular input and in turn projecting inhibition back onto the vestibular relay neurones in the brainstem via its Purkinje cell (P-cell) output (4-11). In outlining this basic circuitry in Fig. 1, I have included only the short latency pathways; polysynaptic and reciprocal inhibitory brainstem pathways have been omitted since they do not have a major bearing on the ideas to be presented here. However, one omission which is very relevant to the later discussions is a mossy fibre input to the flocculus which originates in the vestibular nuclei (12-14); I shall refer to this important projection

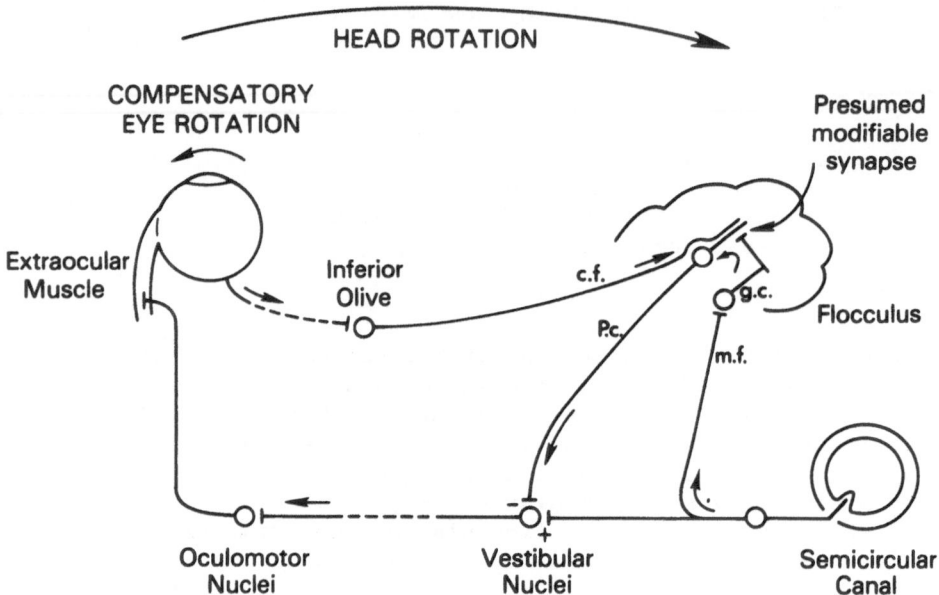

FIGURE 1. A simplified diagram emphasizing the flocculus as an
    inhibitory side-loop of the main vestibulo-ocular pathway,
    receiving a mossy fibre (m.f.) - granule cell (g.c.) primary
    vestibular afferent input and in turn projecting inhibition
    back onto the relay neurones in the vestibular nuclei through
    its Purkinje cell (P.c.) output. Also shown is the visually-
    driven climbing fibre (c.f.) input from the inferior olive,
    an essential element in Ito's hypothetical model for long-
    term adaptive control of the VOR. Ito suggests that activity
    in the c.f. pathway denotes an error in the VOR and, if per-
    sistent, causes a gradual change in the efficacy of the g.c.
    input to the P-cell which will adjust the inhibitory contri-
    bution from the flocculus until the overall VOR gain is once
    again appropriate.

later but for present purposes it can be safely ignored. It is
unfortunate in the light of our current concern with the primate
flocculus, that most of the experiments on which this circuitry is
based were done on the cat and the rabbit; there is some small
consolation from the fact that the little information we do have
about the monkey is at least consistent with this general picture
(15,16).

Like P-cells elsewhere in the cerebellum those in the flocculus
also receive inputs through climbing fibres which originate in the
inferior olive, and there is now abundant evidence that in the cat
(17) and the rabbit (18-22) some of these carry visual information.
Climbing fibres act directly on the P-cell, generating so-called
"complex" spikes (CS's) which are different in form from the
"simple" spikes (SS's) which result from mossy fibre-granule cell
excitation (23). However, while maintained discharge rates of P-
cell SS's are usually high (often exceeding 100/s), those of CS's
are always curiously low (1/s is typical). It seems unlikely that
the climbing fibres, with their sluggish firing rates, could make
any significant contribution to ongoing processes such as the
visual feedback stabilization of the eyes (though this is disputed
by some authors (24,25)), and their functional role remains pole-
mical. A promising suggestion which has recently excited considerable interest, is that the climbing fibres exert some long-term
adaptive influence on transmission through the mossy fibre pathway,
which is the main thoroughfare for on-line information transfer
through the floccular cortex (26-28).

ADAPTIVE CONTROL OF THE VESTIBULO-OCULAR REFLEX (VOR)

The function of the VOR is to help maintain a stable retinal
image during head turns by generating compensatory eye movements
which offset the effects of the head rotations. However, the VOR
operates essentially as a rapid, open-loop, control system, the
labyrinth sensing the head rotation and providing the signals to
initiate compensatory eye movements without the benefit of immediate feedback to indicate the adequacy of those movements (see Fig.
2). Yet, in the rhesus monkey, for example, the VOR achieves a
gain (eye rotation/head rotation) close to unity (29,30), so that
when the monkey turns its head to one side, its eyes rotate almost
an equal amount in the opposite direction even in total darkness.
This raises the question of how the system establishes and maintains appropriate performance levels: essentially, the problem is
one of calibration. No "internal" source of feedback can diagnose
such problems and, in the final analysis, only vision can document
the stability of the retinal image and thereby adduce the adequacy
of the compensatory eye movements coupled to head turns -- persistent image slip signifies the need for a VOR gain adjustment. (In
the light there is, of course, a second ocular stabilization
mechanism working in parallel with the VOR -- the optokinetic

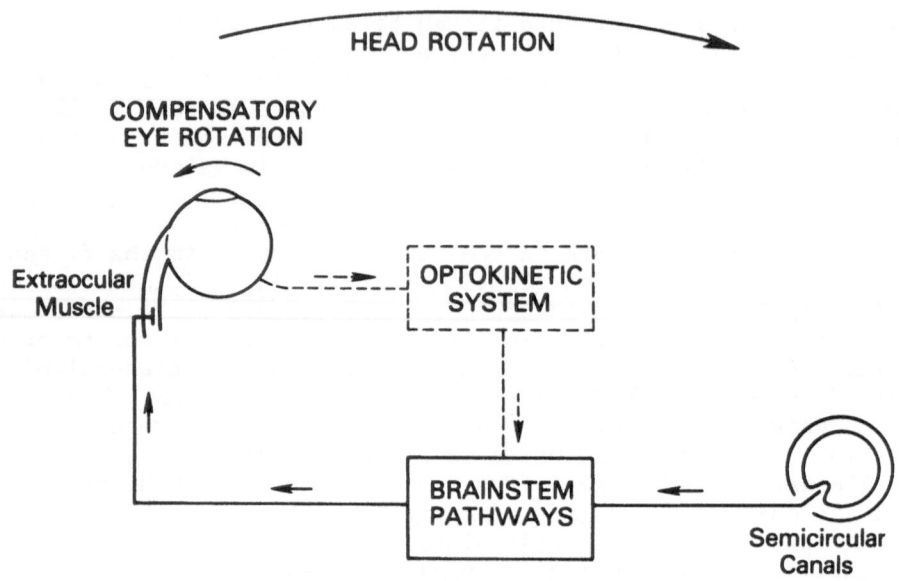

FIGURE 2. The two major systems responsible for retinal image
    stability: the open-loop vestibulo-ocular reflex (fast),
    and the closed-loop optokinetic system (slow).

system -- which operates as a negative, velocity feedback control
system, responding to slippage of the retinal image (31)). Should
the vestibulo-ocular reflex fail to produce complete stability,
then this second system is on hand to reduce the residual retinal
image slip (see Fig. 2). However, extensive dependence on this
visual feedback is a poor substitute for an appropriate VOR because
it is so slow; the VOR, with its inertial receptor and minimal
synaptic delays, is a whole order of magnitude faster than the
optokinetic system, which, in any case, does not even come into
operation until retinal image slip is already under way. An added
advantage of a non-visual mechanism for maintaining ocular stability, and probably one particularly important in the evolution of
the VOR, is that it continues to function in poor luminance condi-

tions. Clearly, there is much to be gained by arranging for the
VOR to carry the main burden of maintaining ocular stability with
minimal immediate dependence on vision, but this requires that the
VOR be appropriately calibrated.

It is now clear that the VOR is modifiable and undergoes
adaptive changes when the visual input normally associated with
head turns is disturbed. Thus, when cats (32,33), monkeys (34),
or human subjects (35) wear dove prism spectacles which reverse
the visual input, the gain of their VOR falls dramatically within
a few days and, in some cases, shows a partial reversal with more
prolonged experience (32, 36). Likewise, telescopic spectacles,
which can be used to magnify or diminish the visual input, when
worn for a few days bring about corresponding increases or decreases
in VOR gain (30, 37). These changes in the VOR are clearly adaptive, operating always to improve stability of the retinal image.
It seems reasonable to assume that this adaptive capability reflects
a continuing need for the VOR to be able to survive the vicissitudes
of normal day-to-day wear and tear over the allotted span of
three-score years and ten or whatever, and does not exist solely
to deal with some chance encounter with spectacles.

Ito (28) was the first to clearly enunciate how the inhibitory
loop of the VOR which incorporates the flocculus might constitute
a variable gain element which could maintain suitable performance
levels within the system. Marr (27) and Albus (26), working
independently, had earlier followed up Brindley's suggestion that
the cerebellum was involved in motor learning (38), by hypothesi-
zing that the synapses between the parallel fibres and P-cells in
the cerebellar cortex were modifiable and invoked the climbing
fibre input as the shaping influence. The major difference between
these two hypotheses was that in Marr's proposal climbing fibre
activation brought about an increase in the efficacy of the parallel
fibre input, while in Albus' model it led to a decrease. Precisely
how the climbing fibre input would bring these changes about was
not specified. In applying the Marr-Albus model, Ito suggested
that the climbing fibres might convey retinal image slip information
to the flocculus to signal the need for a change in the efficacy
of the vestibular parallel fibre input to the P-cell: Ito realized
that the existence of retinal image slip during head turns not
only signalled the need for an adjustment in the gain of the VOR,
but indeed would provide a direct index of the error in the reflex.
This model became even more plausible when it was discovered that
the climbing fibre visual input to the rabbit flocculus was directionally selective (22), with a preference for forward movement
through the visual field (the rabbit having laterally directed
eyes). Furthermore, since this visual input emanates solely from
the ipsilateral eye and the flocculus in the rabbit exerts its
influence only in the ipsilateral horizontal VOR circuitry (8), it
seems to favor Albus' proposal: visual activation of the climbing

fibres would call for a decrease in the inhibitory contribution
from the flocculus.

Others have since invoked Ito's model to explain the adaptive
capability of the VOR (33, 39), and a major current concern is to
establish that the modifiable elements are located in the vestibular
cerebellum. Robinson has recently shown that removal of the
vestibular cerebellum in the cat results in a slight, but permanent,
increase in the gain of the VOR which not even prolonged exposure
to reversing prisms can modify (33). Ito and Miyashita have
claimed that destruction of the climbing fibre input to the flocculus
in the rabbit prevents any long-term adaptive changes in the VOR
(40); unfortunately, the evidence for an adaptive mechanism in
this species is not yet compelling (41).

THE PRIMATE FLOCCULUS

Working with J. H. Fuller, and more recently with B. M. Dow,
I have been studying this system in the awake monkey, using chronic
single unit recording techniques (42). We have examined unit
firing patterns in the flocculus while the animal was subjected to
a variety of visuo-vestibular stimuli designed in part to simulate
the conditions prevailing when the animal first wears magnifying
or reducing spectacles. Our initial concern was to define the
signal processing in the flocculus of the normal monkey, before
proceeding to look for changes associated with long-term exposure
to telescopic spectacles. A convenient and important feature of
single unit studies in the cerebellar cortex is the ability to
distinguish the output P-cells from the other, input elements:
only the P-cells discharge both "complex" and "simple" spikes,
allowing the investigator to make a positive identification of
these output cells (23). Even before we began this study, there
were indications from the work of Lisberger and Fuchs (43) that
the primate flocculus was much more than an appendage of the
vestibulo-ocular pathway. Thus, these workers had already discovered
that the mossy fibre input to the primate flocculus conveyed
oculomotor information, as well as vestibular, and that merely
oscillating the animal often failed to reveal evidence for more
than a very weak vestibular influence on P-cell SS firing (see
Fig. 3A). Indeed, it was only when the animals were called upon
to fixate a target moving in phase with the imposed oscillations
(requiring the animals to use visual tracking to suppress the
normal vestibularly generated compensatory eye movements) that
appreciable modulation of P-cell SS firing -- of presumed vestibular
origin -- was apparent (see Fig. 3B): the vestibular mossy fibre
influence on the P-cell (signalling angular head velocity) was
only evident when the animals' eyes were stationary in their
orbits and not when the VOR was allowed to generate compensatory
eye movements. A possible reason for this seemingly odd finding

first became apparent when Fuller and I found that these same P-cells also discharged SS's in relation to eye velocity -- something which was evident when the monkey tracked moving targets with the head fixed, i.e., eyes moving in the absence of vestibular stimulation (see Fig. 3C). This and subsequent experiments using the simulated telescopic spectacle paradigms showed that the P-cells carry two velocity signals -- relating to head and eyes -- which (1) have the same directional polarity: discharge rates increase with ipsilateral and decrease with contralateral movements, (2) are essentially independent of one another, (3) are often equally weighted, and (4) appear to sum algebraically. Thus, when viewing stationary targets during normal head turns, little SS modulation is apparent in the P-cell output because head and eye velocity are almost equal in amplitude and opposite in direction; hence, the two signals cancel.

An important consequence of this is that the flocculus will contribute little to the overall gain of the VOR in the normal monkey, and brainstem pathways (possibly together with others yet unknown) must accomplish most of the vestibulo-ocular compensation. On the other hand, when the normal monkey is confronted with moving targets, as in the simulated telescopic spectacle paradigms, and must use visual feedback to alter the eye movements coupled to head rotations (i.e., these situations require visual tracking), then the flocculus does make a contribution; as expected, activity in those P-cells with equally weighted head and eye signals (as assessed on the tracking paradigms in Figs. 3B and 3C respectively) always showed a consistently close correlation with gaze velocity -- the sum of orbital eye velocity and head velocity. In these experiments, our highly trained animals usually managed to match their gaze rather closely to the target, and it seemed to Fuller and me that the P-cell SS responses might actually represent a neuronal attempt to model the targets' angular velocity relative to the animal (see Fig. 3). A complete neuronal facsimile of the track target would require a linear sum of three signals: (1) slip velocity of the target's retinal image, (2) eye (orbital) velocity, (3) head velocity. Retinal slip was always very small in our situations but since Fuller and I had observed mossy fibre visual inputs, some of which were directionally selective with the required preference for ipsilateral target movements, we suggested that a visual velocity signal, albeit small, might also be incorporated into P-cell SS firing, thereby completing the velocity profile of the track target. Subsequent recordings suggest that mossy fibre visual inputs are less common than we first thought and gaze velocity is probably more extensively represented than target velocity. This is a difficult issue to investigate, and a rigorous analysis of the information processing will require new experimental paradigms to fully dissociate the vestibular, oculomotor, and visual influences on the P-cell. The existence of

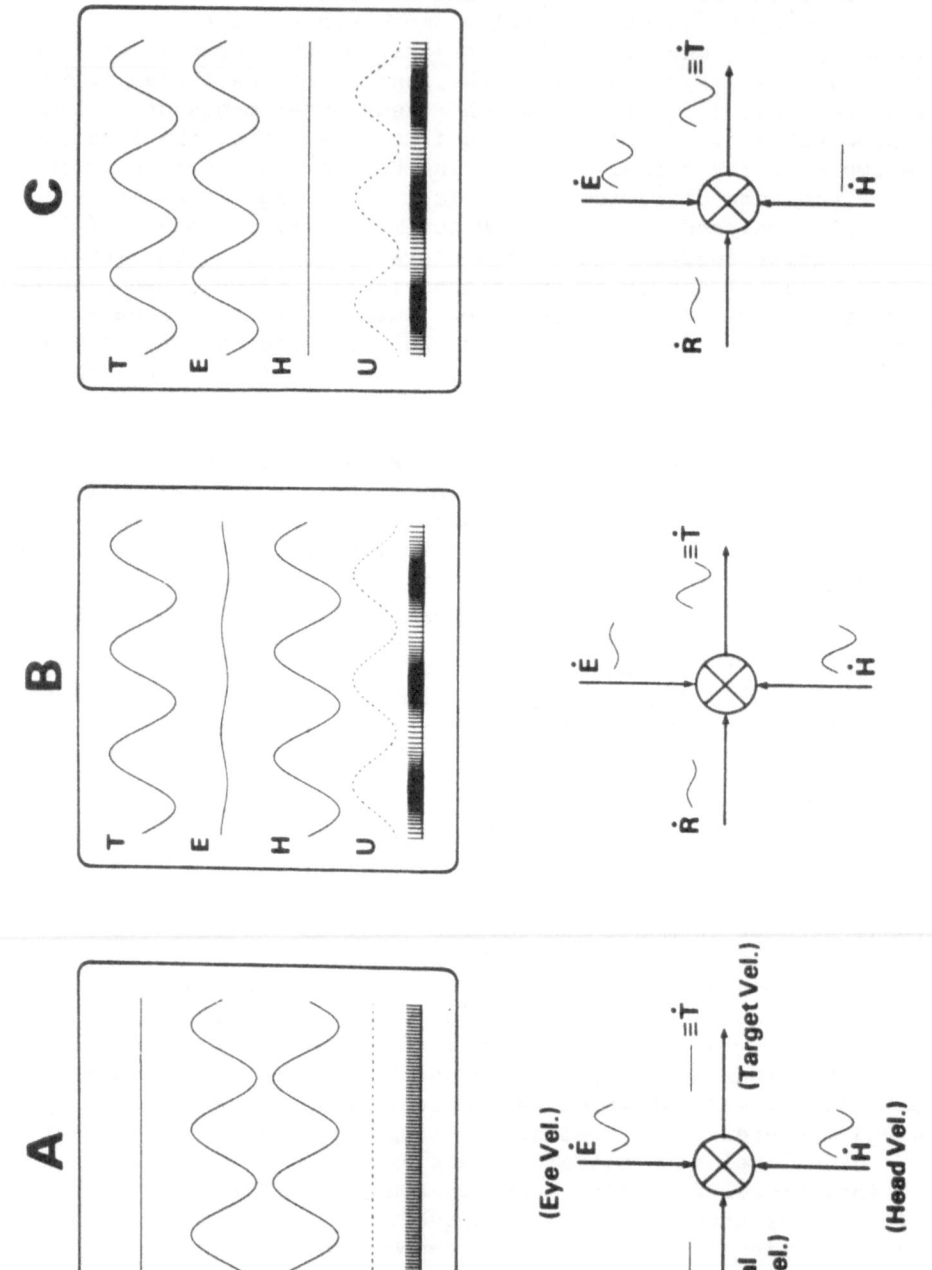

FIGURE 3. A simplified schematic of signal processing in P-cells of the primate flocculus. Above: Idealized representation of the SS discharge characteristics in various tracking paradigms. T, E, and H indicate positions of target, eye and head, respectively; U indicates instantaneous firing rate of the unit with its individual discharges shown beneath. Insets below: Attempt to account for observed P-cell modulation in terms of an algebraic sum of three independent signals — retinal image slip velocity, eye velocity, and head velocity. A: Animal fixates a stationary target while being oscillated, so that eyes and head are always moving at the same rate but in opposite directions. Lack of P-cell modulation is assumed to result from cancellation of the opposing head and eye velocity inputs to the cell; retinal slip input is probably negligible since the VOR, with a gain close to unity, can accomplish the ocular stabilization called for in this paradigm. B: Animal fixates a target moving exactly in phase with the imposed oscillation of the head and hence must use visual tracking to overcome the VOR. Achieved eye velocity is close to zero and P-cell modulation is assumed to derive from the head velocity (vestibular) input, with possibly a small retinal slip contribution. C: The stationary animal now tracks a target moving exactly as in paradigm B. Head velocity is therefore zero and P-cell modulation, which is very similar to that seen in the previous paradigm, is now assumed to derive largely from the eye velocity input, again with possibly a small retinal slip contribution.

oculomotor and visual mossy fibre inputs emphasizes the fact,
mentioned earlier, that the flocculus receives an extensive projection from the vestibular nuclei (and the prepositus hypoglossi -
see Baker this Symposium), in addition to the vestibular primary
afferents featured so prominently in the Ito model. Many of the
eye-movement-related, non P-cell units closely resemble those
recorded in a number of brainstem areas, discharging vigorously in
relation to orbital eye position as well as velocity, often much
like oculomotor motoneurons (44-47). Presumably it is from these
inputs that the P-cell derives its eye velocity signal; the eye
position signals have been largely filtered out and most P-cell
tonic discharges modulate only weakly with changes in static eye
position brought about by saccadic eye movements. A further
intriguing finding is that the maintained firing rates of some
mossy fibre-driven input elements are sensitive only to the fixation
point viewing distance, some increasing with near viewing, others
with distant, and similar tendencies are seen in some P-cell SS
discharges. We do not know if these changes are related to accom-
modation and/or vergence but, interestingly, deficits in convergence
have been noted in cerebellectomized monkeys (48).

These primate studies have revealed little about the information
carried by the climbing fibre input. There is a slight tendency
for some CS discharge rates to modulate out of phase with the SS
discharges (a trend also noted in other species (49)), but there
is nothing to indicate the precise origin of this ultra low frequency
behavior and it has only a minor impact on the high frequency SS
impulse traffic in the P-cell.

The single unit studies in the monkey suggest that the primate
flocculus may have a special role in the on-line stabilization of
retinal images, particularly those of moving, rather than stationary, targets, and Fig. 4 shows our current attempts to model the

FIGURE 4. A tentative signal flow model showing the postulated
            on-line role of the flocculus in the stabilization of the
            retinal image. Loop 1: The major limb of the VOR, confined
            to brainstem pathways. Loop 2: A side limb of the VOR in-
            corporating a variable gain element (G) in the flocculus (cf.
            Ito (28)). Loop 3: Eye velocity (efferent copy) positive
            feedback (cf. Young (51) and Robinson (50)). Loop 4: Visual
            input, providing negative feedback support for tracking θt, θh,
            θe: absolute position of target, head, and eye, respectively.

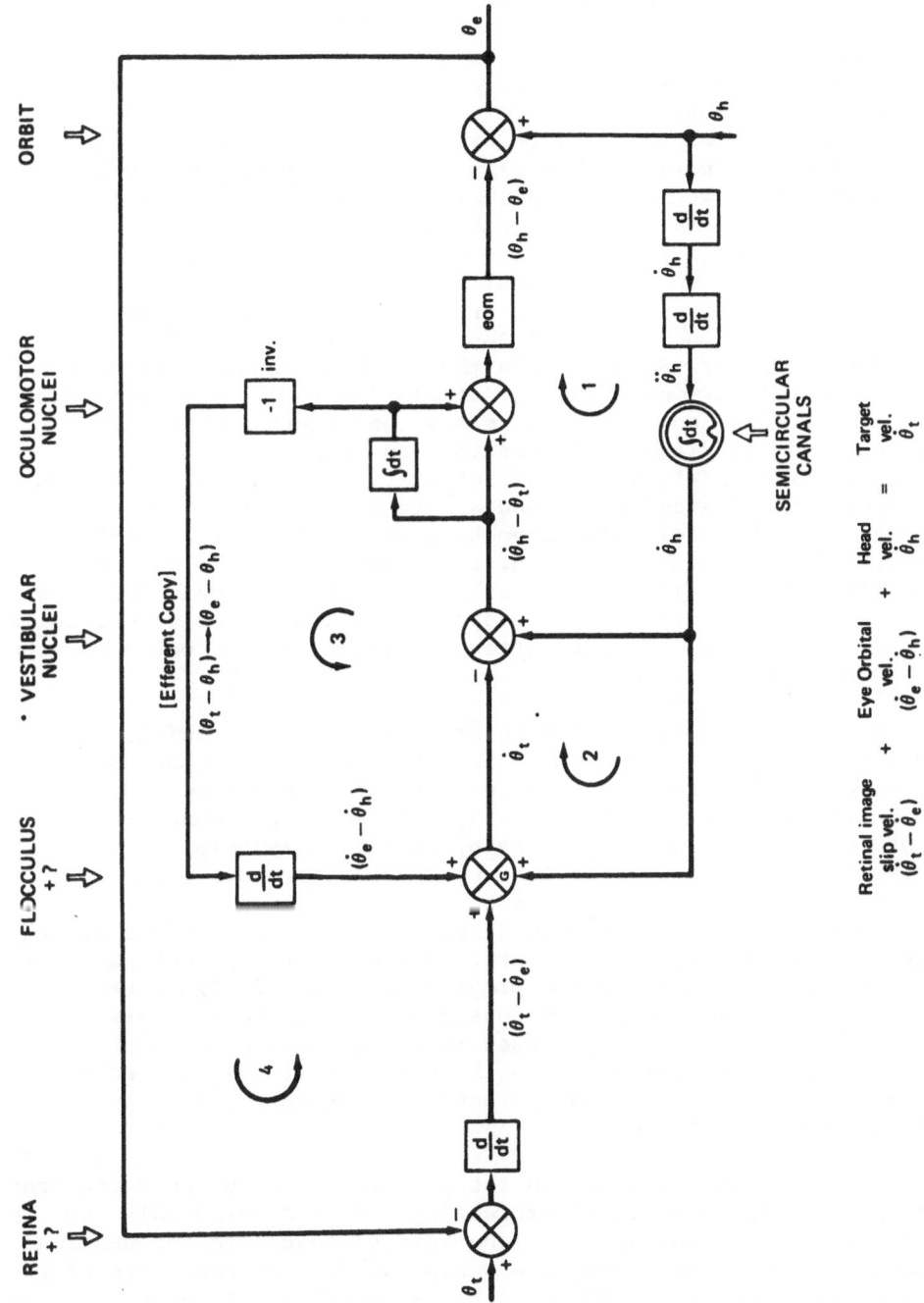

signal processing involved. The first point to note is that it
operates entirely in the velocity domain. The vestibular input to
the P-cell is manifest as a head velocity signal and is assumed to
correspond to Ito's modifiable limb of the VOR (28). The visual
input to the P-cell is assumed to provide negative velocity feedback
support for tracking. The eye velocity component is viewed as a
positive feedback signal derived by differentiation of the incoming
eye position information; this signal would help to sustain tracking
even in the total absence of retinal image slip and features in a
number of theoretical models proposed by others (50, 51). This
positive feedback loop might be responsible for the gradual 'run
away' which occurs in experimental paradigms which exclude the
normal visual 'restraint' (e.g., tracking stabilized images (52)),
and might also be the source of the "second integration" which
Collewijn has proposed to explain the gradual response build-up
during high velocity optokinetic stimulation (53). The continued
operation of this loop in darkness may contribute to the well-
known optokinetic after-nystagmus (54) and might also be one
source of the 'additional neural integration' required to explain
the 'unexpectedly good' low frequency response of the VOR (55).
Deficits in visual following have been reported after cerebel-
lectomy (48) and local lesions of the flocculus (56, 57), and
recent clinical studies have revealed oculomotor pursuit deficits
as well as abnormal vestibular responses in some cases of cerebellar
atrophy (58). However, it is often difficult to rule out brainstem
involvement in the latter.

     Future experiments will also have to consider possible inputs
from neck joint receptors, which have recently been shown to
project to the cat flocculus by both mossy and climbing fibre
routes (14, 59, 60). Such mossy fibre inputs might conceivably
assist combined eye-head tracking by specifically helping to
eliminate those vestibularly induced compensatory eye movements
which would otherwise be coupled to head tracking gestures and
which would hinder, rather than help, ocular pursuit of the moving
target. If these joint inputs arrived over short-latency pathways,
as in the cat, then they might provide the kind of high speed
assistance which is simply not possible through the slow visual
route. None of the paradigms used in the primate experiments
permitted free head movements -- the head was always secured to a
special primate chair and rotary oscillations were passively
imposed upon the whole body.

     The single unit studies in the primate flocculus were concerned
entirely with on-line signal processing and considered only the
immediate effects, and not the long-term consequences, of wearing
telescopic spectacles. From Ito's hypothesis, one would expect to
see long-term adaptive changes in the strength of the head velocity
component of P-cell firing. This is a very specific and testable

prediction and, furthermore, if such changes were found in the P-cells but not in the mossy fibre inputs, then we could conclude that there were indeed modifiable synapses in the cerebellar cortex. Experiments currently under way seek to address this question.

REFERENCES

1. Brodal, A.   Vestibulocerebellar input in the cat: anatomy.
    Prog. Brain Res., 37:315, 1972.

2. Precht, W.   Cerebellar influences on eye movements.   In *Basic
    Mechanisms of Ocular Motility and their Clinical Implications*.
    Lennerstrand, G., and Bach-y-Rita, P., editors.   Oxford,
    Pergamon Press, 1975.

3. Walberg, F.   The vestibular nuclei and their connections
    with the eighth nerve and the cerebellum.   In *The Vestibular
    System*. Naunton, R.F., editor.   New York, Academic Press Inc.,
    1975.

4. Angaut, P., and Brodal, A.   The projection of the "vestibulo-
    cerebellum" onto the vestibular nuclei in the cat. *Arch.
    Ital. Biol.*, 105:441, 1967.

5. Baker, R., Precht, W., and Llinas, R.   Cerebellar modullatory
    action on the vestibulo-trochlear pathway in the cat. *Exptl.
    Brain Res.*, 15:364, 1973.

6. Brodal, A., and Høivik, B.   Site and mode of termination of
    primary vestibulocerebellar fibres in the cat. *Arch. Ital.
    Biol.*, 102:1, 1964.

7. Fukuda, J., Highstein, S.M., and Ito, M.   Cerebellar inhibi-
    tory control of the vestibulo-ocular reflex investigated in
    rabbit IIIrd nucleus. *Exptl. Brain Res.* 14:511, 1972.

8. Ito, M., Nisimaru, N., and Yamamoto, M.   Specific neural
    connections for the cerebellar control of vestibulo-ocular
    reflexes. *Brain Res.*, 60:238, 1973.

9. Walberg, F., Bowsher, D., and Brodal, A.   The termination of
    primary vestibular fibres in the vestibular nuclei in the
    cat. *J. Comp. Neurol.*, 110:391, 1958.

10. Highstein, S.M.   The organization of the vestibulo-oculomotor
    and trochlear reflex pathways in the rabbit. *Exptl. Brain
    Res.*, 17:285, 1973.

11. Precht, W., and Llinas, R.   Functional organization of the
    vestibular afferents to the cerebellar cortex of frog and
    cat. *Exptl. Brain Res.*, 9:30, 1969.

12. Brodal, A., and Torvik, A.   Über den Ursprung der sekundären
    vestibulocerebellaren Fäsern bei der Katze.   Ein experimentell-
    antomische Studie.   *Arch. Psychiat. Nervenkr.*, 195:550, 1957.

13. Shinoda, Y., and Yoshida, K. Neural pathways from the vesti-
    bular labyrinths to the flocculus in the cat. *Exptl. Brain
    Res.*, 22:97, 1975.

14. Wilson, V. J., Maeda, M., Franck, J. I., and Shimazu, H.
    Mossy fiber neck and second-order labyrinthine projections to
    cat flocculus. *J. Neurophysiol.*, 30:301, 1976.

15. Dow, R. S.: Efferent connections of the flocculonodular lobe
    in Macaca mulatta. *J. Comp. Neurol.*, 68:297, 1938.

16. McMasters, R.E., Weiss, A.H., and Carpenter, M.B. Vestibular
    projections to the nuclei of the extraocular muscles. *Amer.
    J. Anat.*, 118:163, 1966.

17. Simpson, J. I., Precht, W., and Llinas, R. Sensory separation
    in climbing and mossy fiber inputs to cat vestibulocerebellum.
    Pflügers Arch., 351:183, 1974.

18. Alley, K., Baker, R., and Simpson, J. I. Afferents to the
    vestibulo-cerebellum and the origin of the visual climbing
    fibers in the rabbit. *Brain Res.*, 98:582, 1975.

19. Maekawa, K., and Kimura, M. Inhibition of climbing fiber
    responses of rabbit's flocculus Purkinje cells induced by
    light stimulation of the retina. *Brain Res.*, 65:347, 1974.

20. Maekawa, K., and Natsui, T. Climbing fiber activation of
    Purkinje cells in rabbit's flocculus during light stimulation
    of the retina. *Brain Res.*, 59:417, 1973.

21. Maekawa, K., and Simpson, J. I. Climbing fiber responses
    evoked in vestibulocerebellum of rabbit from visual system.
    J. Neurophysiol., 36:649, 1973.

22. Simpson, J. I., and Alley, K. E. Visual climbing fiber input
    to rabbit vestibulocerebellum: a source of direction-specific
    information. *Brain Res.*, 82:302, 1974.

23. Eccles, J. C., Ito, M., and Szentagothai, J. *The Cerebellum
    as a Neuronal Machine*. Springer:N.Y., 1967.

24. Simpson, J. I., and Barmack, N. H. Alterations of vestibulo-
    ocular and optokinetic eye movements following lesions of the
    dorsal cap of the inferior olive in rabbits. *6th Ann. Meeting
    Soc. Neurosci.*, Toronto, p. 102, 1976

25. Hess, D. T., and Barmack, N. H. Multiple unitary activity and microstimulation of the inferior olive in rabbits. *6th Ann. Meeting Soc. Neurosci.,* Toronto, p. 110, 1976.

26. Albus, J. S. A theory of cerebellar function. *Math. Biosc.,* 10:25, 1971.

27. Marr, D. A theory of cerebellar cortex. *J. Physiol.,* 202:437, 1969.

28. Ito, M. Neural design of the cerebellar motor control system. *Brain Res.,* 40:81, 1972.

29. Dichgans, J., Bizzi, E., Morasso, P., and Tagliasco, V. The role of vestibular and neck afferents during eye-head coordination in the monkey. *Brain Res.,* 71:225, 1974.

30. Miles, F. A., and Fuller, J. H.: Adaptive plasticity in the vestibulo-ocular responses of the rhesus monkey. *Brain Res.,* 80:512, 1974.

31. Koerner, F., and Schiller, P. H. The optokinetic response under open and closed loop conditions in the monkey. *Exptl. Brain Res.,* 14:318, 1972.

32. Melvill Jones, G., and Davies, P. Adaptation of cat vestibulo-ocular reflex to 200 days of optically reversed vision. *Brain Res.,* 103:551, 1976.

33. Robinson, D. A. Adaptive gain control of vestibulo-ocular reflex by the cerebellum. *J. Neurophysiol.,* 39:954, 1976.

34. Miles, F. A., and Eighmy, B. B. Unpublished observations, 1976.

35. Gonshor, A., and Melvill Jones, G. Short-term adaptive changes in the human vestibulo-ocular reflex arc. *J. Physiol.,* 256:361, 1976.

36. Gonshor, A., and Melvill Jones, G. Extreme vestibulo-ocular adaptation induced by prolonged optical reversal of vision. *J. Physiol.,* 256;381, 1976.

37. Gauthier, G. M., and Robinson, D. A. Adaptation of the human vestibuloocular reflex to magnifying lenses. *Brain Res.,* 92:331, 1975.

38. Brindley, G. S. The use made by the cerebellum of the information that it receives from sense organs. *Int. Brain Res. Org. Bull.,* 3:80, 1964.

39. Davies, P., and Melvill Jones, G. An adaptive neural model
     compatible with plastic changes induced in the human vestibulo-
     ocular reflex by prolonged optical reversal of vision. *Brain
     Res.*, 103:546, 1976.

40. Ito, M., and Miyashita, Y. The effects of chronic destruction
     of the inferior olive upon visual modification of the hori-
     zontal vestibulo-ocular reflex of rabbits. *Proc. Japan
     Acad.*, 51:716, 1975.

41. Collewijn, H., and Kleinschmidt, H. J. Vestibulo-ocular and
     optokinetic reactions in the rabbit: changes during 24 hours
     of normal and abnormal interaction. In *Basic Mechanisms of
     Ocular Motility and their Clinical Implications,* Lennerstrand,
     G., and Bach-y-Rita, R., editors. Oxford, Pergamon Press,
     1975.

42. Miles, F. A., and Fuller, J. H. Visual tracking and the
     primate flocculus. *Science,* 189:1000, 1975.

43. Lisberger, S. G., and Fuchs, A. F. Response of flocculus
     Purkinje cells to adequate vestibular stimulation in the
     alert monkey: fixation vs. compensatory eye movements.
     Brain Res., 69:347, 1974.

44. Luschei, E. S., and Fuchs, A. F. Activity of brainstem
     neurons during eye movements of alert monkeys. *J. Neurophysiol.*,
     35:444, 1972.

45. Miles, F. A. Single unit firing patterns in vestibular
     nuclei related to voluntary eye movements and passive body
     rotation in conscious monkeys. *Brain Res.*, 71:215, 1974.

46. Keller, E. L., and Daniels, P. D. Oculomotor related interac-
     tion of vestibular and visual stimulation in vestibular
     nucleus cells in alert monkey. *Exptl. Neurol.*, 46:187, 1975.

47. Fuchs, A. F., and Kimm, J. Unit activity in vestibular
     nucleus of the alert monkey during horizontal angular accelera-
     tion and eye movement. *J. Neurophysiol.*, 38:1140, 1975.

48. Westheimer, G., and Blair, S. M. Oculomotor defects in
     cerebellectomized monkeys. *Invest. Ophthalmol.*, 12:618,
     1973.

49. Ferin, M., Grigorian, R. A., and Strata, P. Mossy and climbing
     fibre activation in the cat cerebellum by stimulation of the
     labyrinth. *Exptl. Brain Res.*, 12:1, 1971.

50. Robinson, D. A. Models of oculomotor neural organization.
     In *The Control of Eye Movements*. Bach-y-Rita, P., and Collins,
     C. C., editors. New York: Academic Press Inc, 1971.

51. Young, L. R. Pursuit eye tracking movements. In *The Control
     of Eye Movements*. Bach-y-Rita, P., and Collins, C. C.,
     editors. New York: Academic Press Inc, 1971.

52. Robinson, D. A. The mechanics of human smooth pursuit eye
     movement. *J. Physiol.*, 180:569, 1965.

53. Collewijn, H. An analog model of the rabbit's optokinetic
     system. *Brain Res.*, 36:71, 1972.

54. Krieger, H. P., and Bender, M. B. Optokinetic after-nystagmus
     in the monkey. *E. E. G. Clin. Neurophysiol.*, 8:97, 1956.

55. Skavenski, A. A., and Robinson, D. A. Role of abducens
     neurons in vestibuloocular reflex. *J. Neurophysiol.*, 36:724,
     1973.

56. Takemori, S., and Cohen, B. Loss of visual suppression of
     vestibular nystagmus after flocculus lesions. *Brain Res.*,
     72:213, 1974.

57. Ito, M., Shiida, T., Yagi, N., and Yamamoto, M. The cerebellar
     modification of rabbit's horizontal vestibuloocular reflex
     induced by sustained head rotation combined with visual
     stimulation. *Proc. Japan Acad.*, 50:85, 1974.

58. Zee, D. S., Friendlich, A. R., and Robinson, D. A. The
     mechanism of downbeat nystagmus. *Arch. Neurol.*, 30:227,
     1974.

59. Wilson, V. J., Maeda, M., and Franck, J. I. Input from neck
     afferents to the cat flocculus. *Brain Res.*, 89:133, 1975.

60. Wilson, V. J., Maeda, M., and Franck, J. I. Inhibitory
     interaction between labyrinthine, visual and neck inputs to
     the cat flocculus. *Brain Res.*, 96:357, 1975.

OPTOKINETIC NYSTAGMUS AND OPTOKINETIC AFTER-NYSTAGMUS:

CHARACTERISTICS AND FUNCTIONAL SIGNIFICANCE

Bernard Cohen, Victor Matsuo and Theodore Raphan
Department of Neurology
Mount Sinai School of Medicine
City University of New York
New York, New York 10029

The purpose of this paper is to characterize optokinetic nystagmus (OKN) and optokinetic after-nystagmus (OKAN) of the rhesus monkey. From these data we will suggest how the neural mechanism which produces OKN and OKAN might be organized.

Studies were done on juvenile rhesus monkeys implanted with silver-silver chloride electrodes for recording eye position (Bond & Ho, 1971). The animals had bolts implanted in the skull to hold the head rigidly during testing. Each animal received amphetamine sulphate (0.5 mg/kg), about a half hour before testing to maintain a constant level of alertness. Monkeys sat under an optokinetic drum on a rotating platform. The drum was made of white plastic and was internally lighted, and had 3° diameter black stripes at intervals of 45°. An important aspect of the stimulus was that it filled the animal's visual field. This was accomplished by placing a mirror under the chin of the monkey. The mirror reflected the stripes on the ceiling of the drum and provided a powerful stimulus for inducing OKN. Under these test conditions every animal had OKN which persisted for the duration of stimulation. It was a reflex response which was not dependent on training or on the cooperation of the animal.

What is the significance of the full field rotation and of the OKN which it induces? Ordinarily the entire visual surround rotates when the head is moved. OKN tends to stabilize images on the retina by matching eye velocity to the velocity of the moving surround. Therefore OKN induced by full field stimulation may participate with the vestibular system in compensating for head movement.

Ter Braak (1936) pointed out that if a rabbit rotates at a constant velocity in darkness, compensatory vestibular nystagmus dies away quickly. However, if the rotation is in light, the nystagmus is maintained indefinitely. He attributed the continuation of the nystagmus to the induction of OKN. We have studied this using slow phase velocity as an index of the interaction. If monkeys are rotated in darkness at a constant velocity, per-rotatory nystagmus is induced at the onset of stimulation and post-rotatory nystagmus occurs at the end of stimulation. There is a sudden rise in slow phase velocity at the beginning and end of the steps in angular velocity. Slow phase velocity is maintained for several seconds and then falls gradually over about 20 to 60 seconds. In contrast, if a step in optokinetic drum velocity is given, the velocity of the slow phases of OKN rises to a peak value more slowly, but then is maintained for the duration of the stimulus.

When the optokinetic and vestibular responses are combined, they produce a step change in eye velocity in response to the step change in stimulus velocity (Fig. 1). Moreover, as orginally shown by Ter Braak, at the end of stimulation post-rotatory nystagmus and OKAN, which are oppositely directed, summate and there is little or no post-rotatory nystagmus (Fig. 1, arrow). Thus, OKAN appears to reduce the amount of the post-rotatory vestibular response to prolonged angular head movement in light.

This test paradigm, i.e., simultaneous drum and surround stimulation is useful in establishing a basis for calibration of the EOG. Robinson and Skavenski (1973) showed that in the monkey the gain of the vestibulo-ocular reflex in light is close to unity (Eye velocity/stimulus velocity). That is, the velocity of the slow phases of nystagmus induced by combined optokinetic and vestibular stimuli is close to the difference between platform velocity and surround velocity. If the velocity of the nystagmus generated in response to angular rotation in light is known, it can be compared to the velocity of the response to optokinetic stimulation.

Figure 2 demonstrates that the velocity of slow phases of nystagmus induced by full field rotation (seen at the left) or by full field rotation plus angular rotation (right) both vary linearly between 22 and 90°/sec. The slope and intercept of the lines were the same. Thus, slow phases had the same velocity whether the optokinetic drum moved around the animal or whether the animal itself was moving inside the stationary drum. This demonstrates that full field rotation is a powerful stimulus and in the monkey is capable of driving the eyes at gains close to unity.

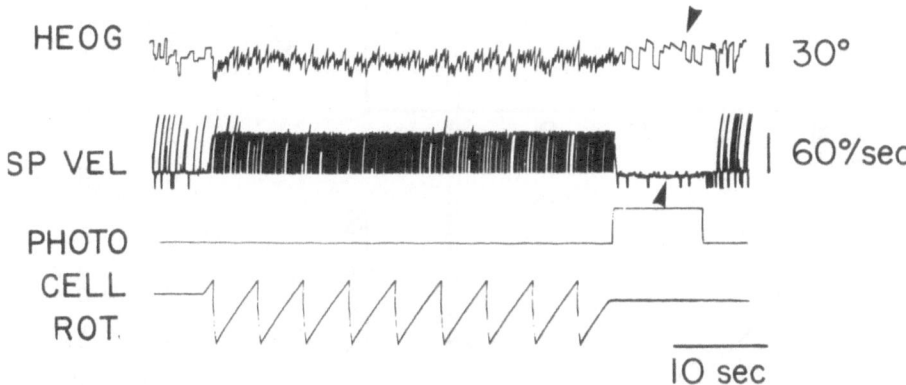

CCW ROTATION (60°/sec)
STATIONARY DRUM

HEOG | 30°

SP VEL | 60°/sec

PHOTO
CELL
ROT.

10 sec

FIGURE 1. Eye movements induced by angular rotation at 60°/sec in light under a stationary drum. Top trace, horizontal EOG (calib. amplitude 30°); second trace, slow phase velocity (calib. 60°/sec); third trace, photocell recording light (down) and darkness (up); fourth trace, platform rotation with each return measuring 360°. At the end of rotation the animal was in darkness for 10 seconds. Note the step change in eye velocity in response to the step change in platform velocity. Note also the very weak post-rotatory nystagmus at the end of rotation.

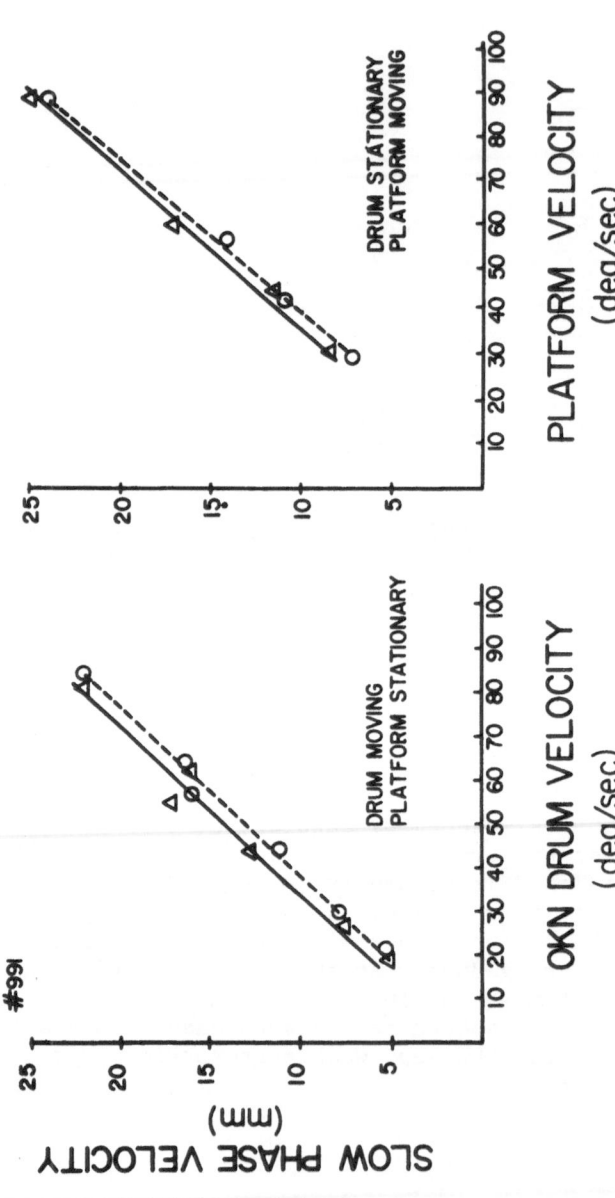

FIGURE 2. Graphs of slow phase eye velocity (ordinate) induced by OKN stimulation (left) and by angular rotation (right) in the light at velocities of 20–90°/sec. Triangles refer to rightward and open circles to leftward nystagmus. The slopes and intercepts of the line were the same for the two stimulus conditions.

We have recently done a thorough analysis of the velocity characteristics of OKN and OKAN induced by full field rotation (Cohen, Matsuo & Raphan, 1977), and some of the highlights of that study will be summarized here. Typical velocity traces during OKN and OKAN of a monkey in response to different velocities of stimulation are shown in Figure 3. In this experiment the animal was sitting in darkness and lights were switched on suddenly while the drum was rotating. Thus the animal was presented with a step change in velocity of the rotating field. In response to this stimulus, there was a sudden rise in slow phase velocity over several beats of nystagmus, followed by a slower rise to the steady state value. Although data are only presented for 29, 62, 90, and 180°/sec, the same sequence of slow and rapid rise was found at lower velocities as well and we take this to be a general phenomenon. Over a range of stimuli up to between 90 and 120°/sec, the ratio between the initial velocity and steady state velocity was about 0.6.

As stimulus velocity increased, the time from onset of stimulation to the steady state was longer. When maximum velocities rose above 90 to 120°/sec, the ensuing nystagmus became more irregular and the velocities varied considerably (Fig. 3, 180°/sec). It is of interest that monkeys were able to follow moving stimuli at slow phase velocities of about 180°/sec in response to full field stimulation. This is considerably faster than following in humans (Grüttner, 1939).

If the lights are left on at the end of optokinetic stimulation, the nystagmus disappears in several seconds. However, if animals are in complete darkness after OKN, OKAN persists for periods of 20 to 60 seconds (Krieger & Bender, 1956; and Fig. 3). The persistance of OKAN is remarkable because nothing has moved during stimulation except the visual field and the eyes. This suggests that a storage mechanism or "integrator" had been activated by the visual stimulus, which continues to discharge in the subsequent period of OKAN.

The charge and discharge characteristics of this storage mechanism were studied. To determine "charge time" the drum was rotated around a monkey while it was sitting in darkness. The drum was illuminated for short periods (0.1–10 seconds), and peak OKN velocities achieved during the light period as well as the peak velocity of the subsequent OKAN were measured. Since EOG gain is affected by darkness, these experiments were done just after the animal was given a 60°/sec calibrating stimulus, and OKAN was observed for not more than 10 seconds after the end of OKN. OKAN and OKN slow phase velocities were normalized in relation to the velocity induced by the 60°/sec stimulus. As noted, this velocity was presumed to be close to the actual velocity of the drum.

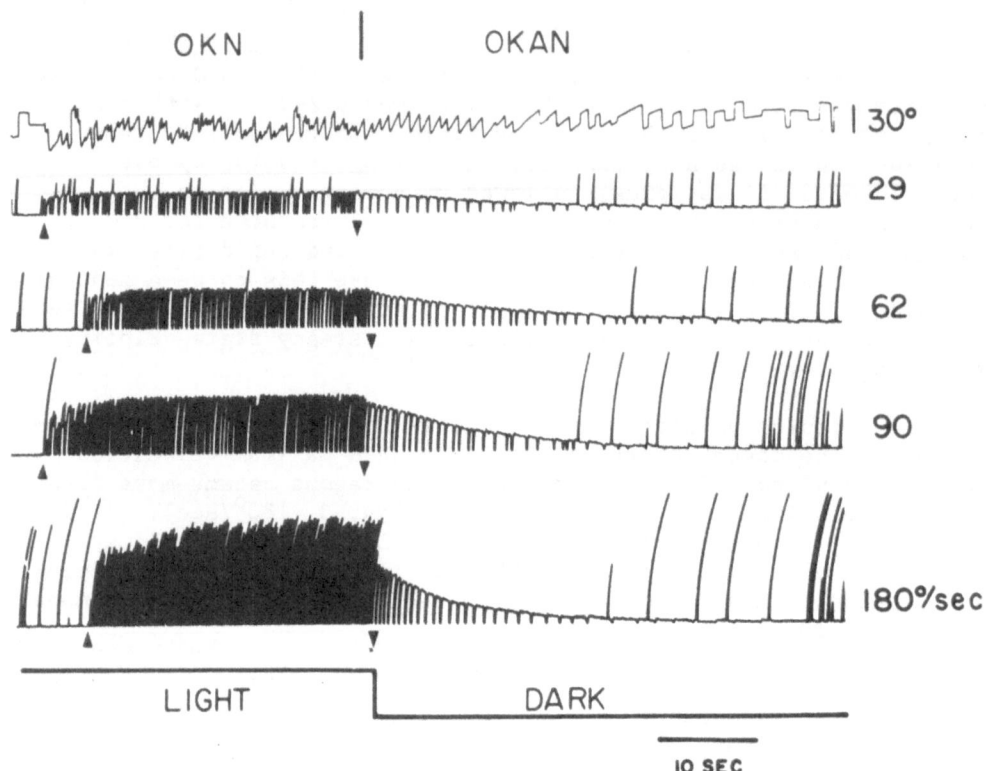

FIGURE 3. Slow phase velocity of OKN and OKAN induced by full
field rotations of 29° to 180°/sec. The horizontal EOG
(calib. 30°) and slow phase velocity traces are both shown
for the stimulus of 29°/sec. For other stimulus velocities
only the slow phase velocity trace is shown. During OKN
there was an initial rapid rise in velocity followed by a
slower rise to a steady state level. At the onset of OKAN
there was an initial fall in slow phase velocity, followed
by a slower decline to zero. The rate of decline during OKAN
increased with increases in stimulus velocity. The calibration
for the velocity traces is given by the amplitude of the steady
state OKN velocity, which is assumed to be approximately equal
to that of the stimulus velocity (see text).

Figure 4 shows a typical example of the response to a short period of optokinetic stimulation. Note the rapid rise in slow phase velocity at the onset of OKN followed by a much lower velocity of OKAN. This shows that the mechanisms responsible for OKN and OKAN are not identical.

At the onset of OKAN the drop in velocity was striking after brief periods of stimulation (Fig. 4). However, if longer durations of stimulation were used, OKAN velocities approached the velocity of the preceding OKN (Fig. 3). The duration of stimulation necessary to maximize OKAN velocity was the same as the duration necessary to produce steady state OKN. This suggests a close correspondence between the processes responsible for producing the slow rise in OKN and those producing OKAN.

An additional aspect of OKAN which was investigated was the rapid decline of OKAN slow phase velocity in light. If the lights were left on at the end of OKN, OKAN slow phase velocity declined to zero in several seconds. At the end of this period if the animal was again put in darkness, OKAN did not return. This demonstrates that the storage mechanism responsible for OKAN had been discharged by visual fixation.

The time course of discharge of the OKAN mechanism was tested by giving short periods of fixation and noting recovery of OKAN velocity in the subsequent period of darkness. Durations of fixation necessary to completely discharge the OKAN mechanism were 2.5 to 3 seconds in several monkeys. A typical example of a partial discharge of the OKAN mechanism is shown in Fig. 5. Slow phase velocity would normally have fallen along a course close to the dotted line. During OKAN however, the lights were turned on for 0.4 sec. with the drum stationary. At the end of this period of fixation when the animal was again in darkness, OKAN became more vigorous, but its velocity was less than the velocity observed when there was no period of fixation. That is, the short period of fixation had caused a partial discharge of the storage mechanism responsible for OKAN.

From the preceding data we postulate that there are rapid pathways from the visual system to the oculomotor system which drive the eyes at the onset of OKN to some fraction of the total stimulus velocity. The fact that the ratio of initial to steady state velocity of OKN is similar for all stimulus velocities up to 90–120°/sec is taken to mean that OKN is generated similarly by every stimulus velocity in this range. The finding that the slow rise during OKN and the charge of the OKAN mechanism are accomplished over the same period of time is taken to mean that the same central storage mechanism or integrator is responsible for both.

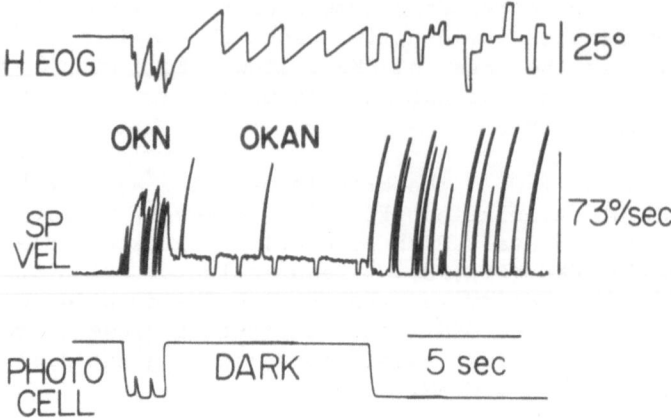

FIGURE 4. Incomplete charge of OKAN mechanism by full field rotation. Stimulation for a brief period (1.8 sec) at 73°/sec induced OKN and OKAN. The stationary OKN drum was lighted 10 seconds after the onset of OKAN terminating the trial. Note the abrupt drop in slow phase velocity at the onset of OKAN.

73%S RT. OKN

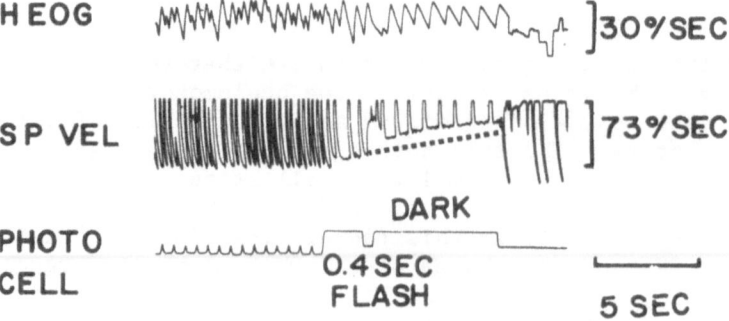

FIGURE 5. Effect of short (.4 sec) period of fixation on OKAN.

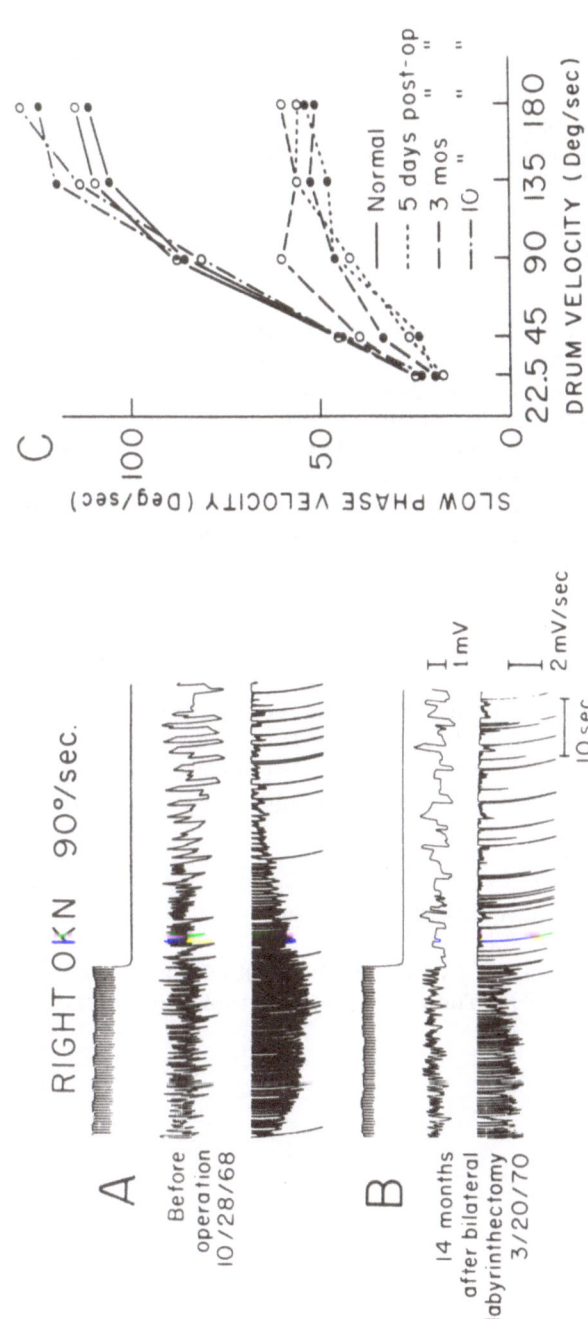

FIGURE 6. OKN and OKAN before (A) and after (B) bilateral labyrinthectomy in monkey 707. Top trace, photocell output showing passage of drum stripes. Stimulus velocity 90°/sec. Second trace, horizontal EOG; third trace, slow phase velocity. The EOG was recorded with platinum needle electrodes. The animal was in darkness at the end of stimulation. Note the absence of a slow rise in OKN slow phase velocity and the loss of OKAN after operation (B). (From Fig. 8, page 16, Uemura & Cohen, Acta Otolaryng. (Stockh.), Suppl 315, 1973). C, Slow phase velocity as a function of stimulus velocity before (solid lines) and after bilateral labyrinthectomy in monkey 919. For 3–6 months after operation OKN slow phase velocity saturated at about 60°/sec. (From Fig. 2, pp. 90, Cohen, Uemura & Takemori, Equilibrium Research 3: 1973).

It was predicted that if the integrator were inactivated,
there would be no slow rise in OKN velocity, only a rapid rise.
Such data were obtained in experiments on the vestibular system
(Uemura & Cohen, 1973). After bilateral labyrinthectomy, OKAN was
permanently abolished. The loss of OKAN suggests that the storage
mechanism responsible for OKAN had been inactivated. If correct,
then the mechanism responsible for the slow rise in OKN velocity
to the steady state level should also be absent. Moreover, the
highest attainable OKN velocity should be only about 60% of the
steady state velocity reached before operation, being due primarily
to activation of the direct pathways.

Figure 6 shows data from a monkey before and after bilateral
labyrinthectomy. Before the operation (Fig. 6A), OKN was characterized by a rapid and slow rise in slow phase velocity and by
typical OKAN. After bilateral labyrinthectomy (Fig. 6B), the
animal no longer had OKAN; its OKN was irregular and no longer had
a slow rise to a peak steady state value. In agreement with the
above prediction the maximum slow phase velocity during OKN was
about 60% of that recorded before operation in response to a
similar stimulus.

These data provide evidence for the presence of a storage
mechanism acting during OKAN. This storage mechanism might help
balance long duration post-rotatory vestibular responses, help
maximize slow phase velocity during OKN, and regularize eye velocities
during nystagmus induced by full field rotation. Monitoring the
activity in these integrators could also be important for perceiving
self-motion during angular head movement (Brandt & Dichgans,
1972).

ACKNOWLEDGEMENTS

Supported by: NIH Research Grant, NINCDS 00294 and CUNY
Research, Faculty Award 11058. Theodore Raphan was supported by
NINCDS Fellowship NS052970.

REFERENCES

Bond, H.W, and Ho, P.   Solid miniature silver-silver chloride
    electrodes for chronic implanation. *Electroenceph. Clin.
    Neurophysiol.*, 28:206-208, 1970.

Brandt, T., and Dichgans, J.   Circularvektion, optische Pseudo-
    orioliseffekte und optokinetisher Nachnystagmus. *Albrecht v.
    Graefes Arch. klin. exp. Ophthal.*, 184:42-57, 1972.

Cohen, B., Matsuo, V. and Raphan, T.   Quantitative analysis of the
    velocity characteristics of optokinetic nystagmus and opto-
    kinetic after-nystagmus, in press. *J. Physiol.*, 1977.

Gruttner, R.   Experimentelle Untersuchungen uber den optokinetischen
    Nystagmus. *Zeitschrift fur Sinnesphysiol.*, 68:1-48, 1939.

Robinson, D.A., and Skavenski, A.   Role of abducens neurons in
    vestibulo-ocular reflex. *J. Neurophysiol.*, 36:724-738, 1973.

Ter Braak, J.W.G.   Untersuchungen uber optokinetischen Nystagmus.
    Arch. Neerl. Physiol., 21:309-376, 1936.

Uemura, T. and Cohen, B.   Effects of vestibular nuclei lesions on
    vestibulo-ocular reflexes and posture in monkeys. *Acta oto-
    laryngol. Suppl.*, 315:1-71, 1973.

THE ROLE OF THE BRAIN STEM RETICULAR FORMATION IN EYE MOVEMENT

CONTROL

Edward L. Keller
Department of Electrical Engineering and Computer Sciences
and the Electronics Research Laboratory
University of California
Berkeley, California

A previous review (Cohen and Henn, 1972b) has summarized the past work on oculomotor relations of the brain stem reticular formation including information from lesion studies, electrical stimulation, and field potential analysis. These studies as a whole support the hypothesis that this region of the reticular formation, and in particular the medial pontine reticular formation (PRF), is the location of the immediate supranuclear neural structures responsible for generating conjugate horizontal rapid eye movements (saccades and the quick-phase movements of nystagmus). This review will concentrate on the additional support for this view that has accumulated in the form of single-unit recordings in alert animals, electrophysiological studies of synaptic connections, and detailed neuroanatomical tracing techniques. In addition some new data on functional interconnections of the PRF with the superior colliculus (SC), a higher visual-motor control center also implicated in the generation of saccades, will be presented.

The specific anatomic locations emphasized in this review correspond to the medial regions of the nucleus reticularis pontis oralis and caudalis and the rostral portion of nucleus giganto cellularis in the cat. Homologus cellular groups are found in the primate (Olszewski, 1954) although the rostro-caudal delimitations between nuclear groups are less clear. The areas under consideration thus include portions of the medial medullary reticular formation as well as the pontine RF. Nevertheless, the area will be referred to simply as the PRF. More rostral reticular areas including the mesencephalic RF will not be considered in the present review.

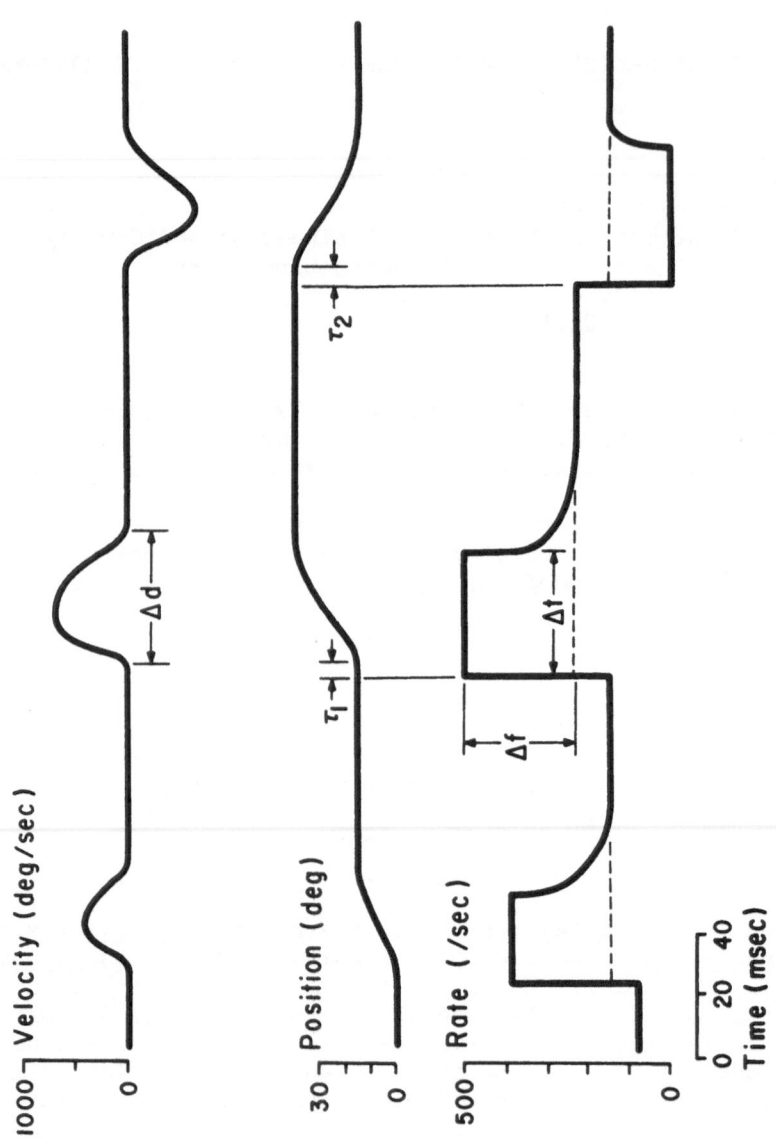

SUPRANUCLEAR SIGNALS REQUIRED BY OCULOMOTOR NEURONS

A logical starting point for the discussion of the supranuclear organization is a brief review of the discharge patterns observed in oculomotor neurons during rapid eye movements and the intervening periods of fixation.

It is now generally accepted that saccades are produced by a pulse-step change in motoneuron discharge rate (Robinson and Keller, 1972). All motoneurons participate in a manner similar to that shown in Fig. 1 for schematic horizontal eye movements. When innervating an agonist (two saccades on the left) each motoneuron discharges a burst of spikes that slightly precedes (τ_1) the onset of the saccade and that is maintained for a duration (Δt) similar to the duration (Δd) of the saccade. Accompanying each such saccadic pulse is a smaller step change in motoneuron firing rate that is maintained in a remarkably constant manner throughout the next period of steady fixation. The innervation pattern when the muscle innervated is the antagonist (saccade on the right) is a mirror image of that present in the agonist. A brief interval of discharge cessation (negative pulse) slightly precedes (τ_2) the start of the movement and continues for the duration of the saccade. There is also a step change in motoneuron discharge to the lower steady level associated with the new position of eye fixation. Although the quantitative parameters describing the relative size of the pulse (Δf) and envelope of its shape vary in a continuous manner across the population of motoneurons (Henn and Cohen, 1973), this description fits in a qualitative manner the observed discharge pattern of all motoneurons.

Quantitative measures have been made of a number of these parameters which will be cited here for their relevance in determining the nature of the required supranuclear signals. The pulse in motoneuron activity leads (τ_1 and τ_2) the onset of eye movement by about 5-8 msec and is complete at about the same interval preceding the end of the movement. Larger saccades are made with

---

FIGURE 1. Typical oculomotor neuron discharge behavior during saccades and fixation. Middle trace: horizontal eye position; Upper trace: eye velocity for the three saccadic movements shown; Lower trace: motoneuron instantaneous discharge rate. The dashed lines illustrate the step change in firing rate associated with the change in eye position during each saccade. See text for a discussion of the remaining symbols.

higher eye velocities (upper trace, Fig. 1), and this results for
the most part from a larger pulse (Δf) of motoneuronal activity.
There is a graded variation in this behavior with some motoneurons
showing a much more dramatic increase in Δf in correlation with
higher peak saccadic velocity (Robinson, 1970).

Since oculomotor neurons appear to be free of recurrent or axon
collaterals (Sasaki, 1963), and also are not affected by short-
latency feedback from orbital proprioceptors (Keller and Robinson,
1971), the final common path can be considered an open-loop system
in which the shape of the discharge frequency envelope of motoneurons must be generated by a similar (in time) supranuclear
input. Membrane properties of the motoneurons themselves may alter
to some degree the dynamics of this signal transfer (Barmack,
1974), but the basic pulse and the step signal must be generated in
some supranuclear structure. Indeed, intracellular recordings in
oculomotor neurons during induced nystagmus show that for each rapid
eye movement, the pulse of activity in the agonist results from a
burst of synaptic EPSPs and the pause in antagonist results from a
burst of IPSPs (Maeda et al., 1972; Baker and Berthoz, 1974).

SINGLE-NEURON ACTIVITY IN THE PRF

Guided by this knowledge of the required supranuclear signals
a number of recording studies have been made in the PRF of alert,
behaving monkeys (Sparks and Travis, 1971; Cohen and Henn, 1972a;
Luschei and Fuchs, 1972). The attempt in these early studies was to
classify the types of unit behavior seen in the PRF during saccades
and for fixations at a range of eye positions. The variety of unit
responses recorded in this area were classified into burst cells,
units which discharged high-frequency bursts of spikes preceding and
during rapid eye movements; pause cells, units which ceased firing
completely during saccades but discharged at steady rates during
periods of fixation; and tonic cells, units which fired at steady
rates correlated with eye position during periods of fixation. A
group of neurons which discharged at rates proportional to eye
position in some preferred direction (on-direction) but which also
discharged bursts of spikes or were inhibited during saccades in the
on and off-direction respectively formed a subdivision of the basic
tonic classification. These cells, which were named burst-tonic
units, thus closely resemble oculomotor neurons. Data reported on
this type of cell raised the possibility that the pulse and the step
signal were already preassembled at a supranuclear level before
projection to oculomotor neurons. Similar cell responses have now
been recorded in the vestibular nuclei (Miles, 1974; Fuchs and Kimm,
1975; Keller and Daniels, 1975) and in the MLF (Davis-King et al.,
1975; and Pola, 1975).

Burst units. In a more recent paper Keller (1974) focused attention on one particular type of PRF burst cell, called the medium-lead burster, which initiated an extremely high-frequency (600–1000 spike/sec) burst just prior (on average 3 msec) to the average initiation time of motoneurons' saccadic burst or pause. For ipsilateral horizontal movements the average duration of the high-frequency burst just equaled that of the average motoneuron's burst or pause for the same size eye movement. A typical example of this type of unit is shown in Fig. 2. When the eye movement was in an oblique direction, the unit continued to discharge a burst which had the same duration as the ipsilateral horizontal component of the movement. These units did not discharge, or showed at most a few irregular discharges, if the movement was purely vertical or had a contralateral horizontal component. The intraburst frequency of the burst was monotonically related to the velocity (and hence size) of the movement, as shown in Fig. 3. Thus these units could provide the complete supranuclear control signal required to generate the saccadic behavior of the horizontally acting oculomotor neurons.

An alternative parameter describing the coding present in these burst cells is the number of discharges in the burst. When the number of discharges in the bursts were plotted as functions of saccade size a very linear relationship resulted (Keller, 1974; Henn and Cohen, 1976). These results show that in an informational coding sense either duration of the burst or number of spikes in the burst of this type of supranuclear neuron could be considered to be equivalent. However, in terms of direct generation of the duration of motoneurons' saccadic burst, the duration of supranuclear cells' bursts seems to be the more probable control mechanism. In addition the higher medium-lead burst unit frequency observed during larger saccades seems to be an adequate explanation for the higher burst rate of motoneurons and hence higher eye velocities for the larger movements. This type of neuron constituted only about 7% of the total sample of neurons studied in the PRF (Keller, 1974). Cohen and Henn (1976) have described a similar group of neurons active for horizontal saccades and another group of related neurons whose discharge has a duration which approximately equals the duration of the vertical component of the movement. Together these two types of neuron constituted about 30% of their sample of PRF units. Their results suggest that signals controlling both the horizontal and vertical movers of the eye may lie in the PRF. This would not be consistent with the results of experiments which show only deficits in the horizontal gaze system following PRF lesions (Cohen et al., 1968). One possible explanation might be that supranuclear neurons controlling the motoneurons for vertical eye movements are distributed bilaterally in the PRF while those controlling each direction of horizontal movement are exclusively (Keller, 1974) or predominately (Henn and Cohen, 1976) distributed on only one side. The

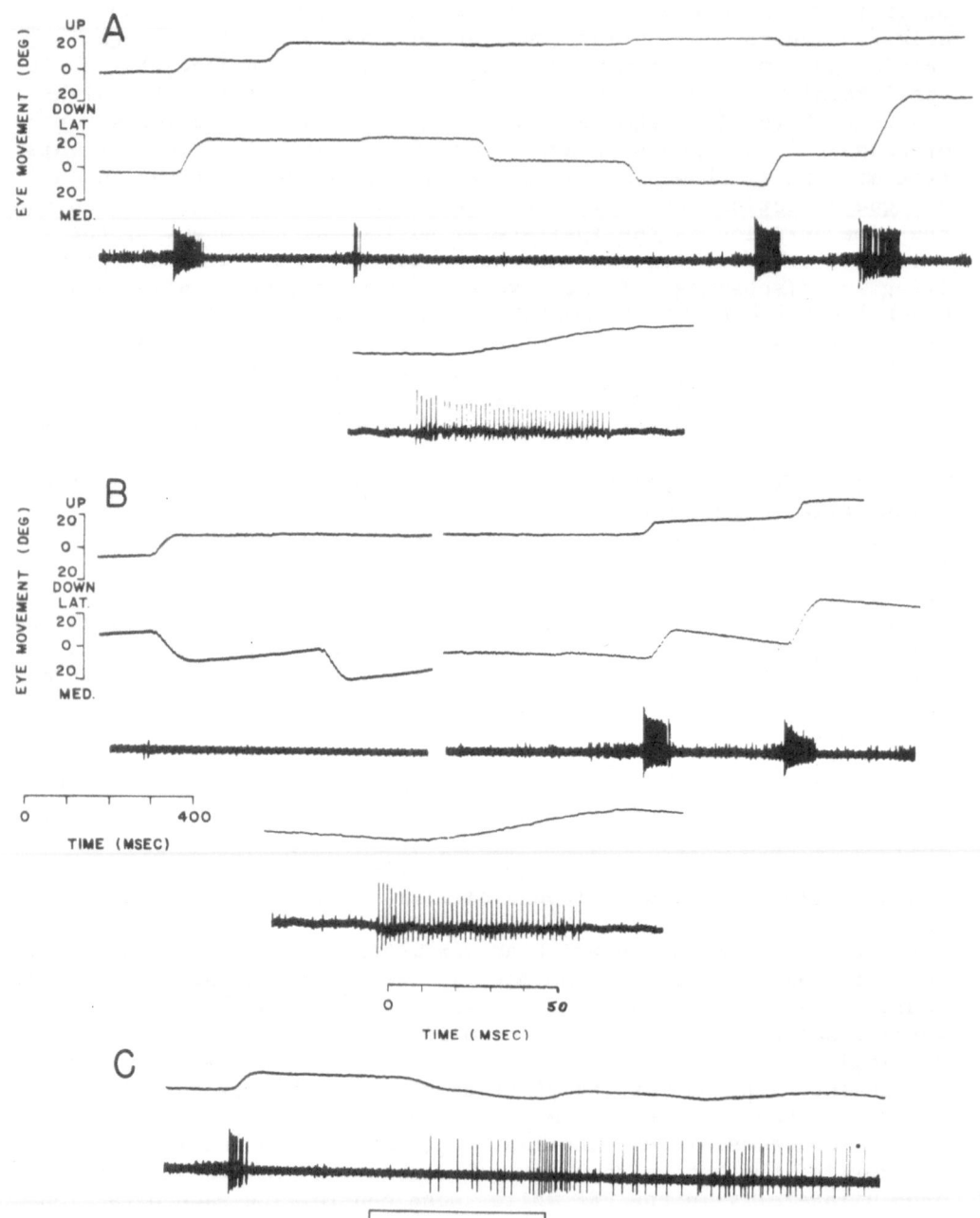

FIGURE 2. Activity of a medium-lead burst unit recorded in the
   right PRF during saccadic eye movements (A), the quick-phase
   movements of rotationally induced vestibular nystagmus (B),
   slow drifting eye movements of the initial stages of slip (C).
   In A and B upper trace is vertical and middle trace is
   horizontal eye position. The time calibration for both shown
   in B. In C only horizontal eye position is shown with the
   same calibration as in A and B. Insets in A and B are high-
   speed records of one horizontal rapid eye movement and
   associated unit activity. Time calibration in C is 0.5msec.
   All eye movements measured on the right eye.

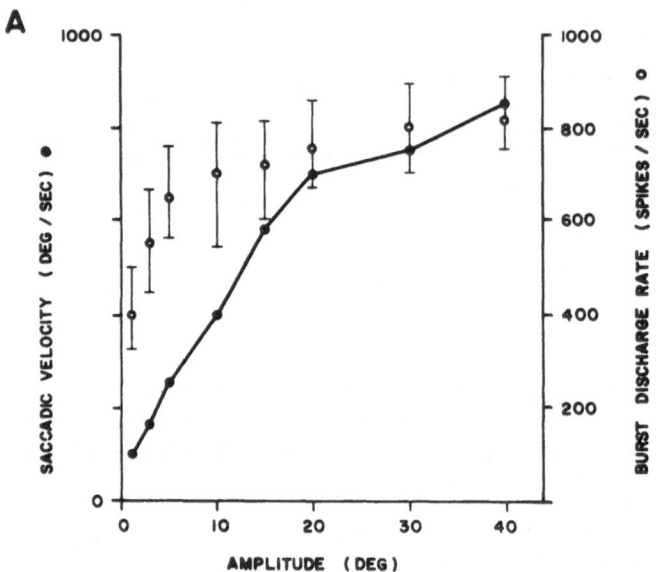

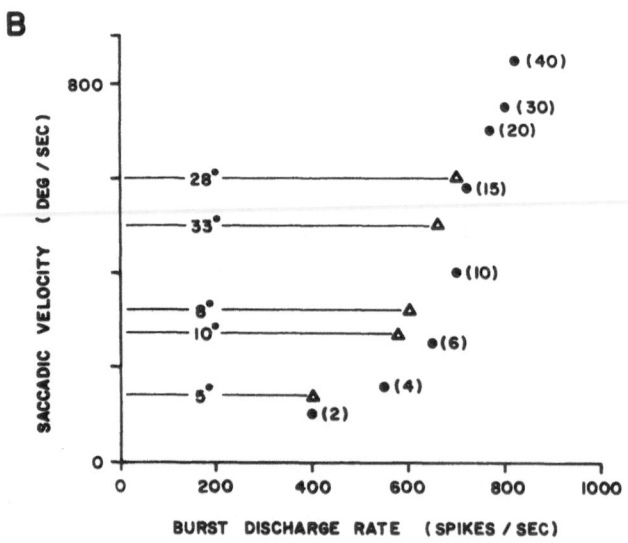

FIGURE 3. A: The relationship between saccadic amplitude and
    maximum saccadic velocity (filled circles). Each point
    represents the mean from at   least 10 saccadic movements of
    each size. Also shown is at   relationship between saccade
    size and the associated burst frequency for medium-lead
    burst units (open circles). Each point represents the grand
    mean of the maximum burst rates associated with the 10 saccades
    of each size for 16 PRF units (the bars are ranges of the
    means). B: The means (burst rate and velocity) from A re-
    plotted to show the relationship between intraburst firing
    frequency and saccadic velocity (filled circles). The numbers
    in parentheses are the amplitudes of the saccades associated
    with each point. The triangles show maximum saccadic velocity
    and associated burst rate for several abnormally slow saccades
    of the size shown on the interruped horizontal lines. Note
    that burst rate continues to code saccadic velocity for these
    slow movements.

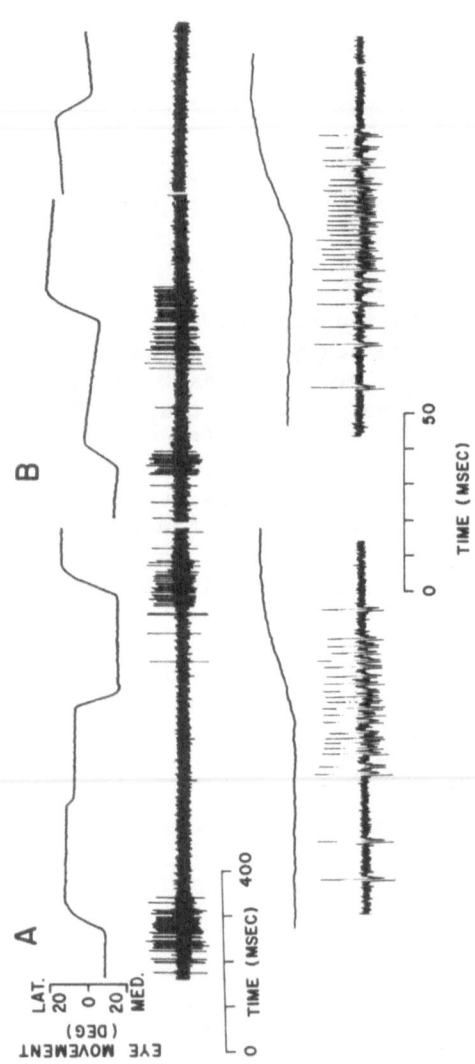

FIGURE 4. Activity of a long-lead burst unit during saccadic eye
movements (A) and the quick-phase movement of vestibular
nystagmus (B). Eye movement and time calibration of nystagmus
(B). Eye movement and time calibration the same in A and B.
Only the horizontal component of eye position shown. Insets
below A and B are high-speed records of one horizontal rapid
eye movement of each type and associated unit activity.

reported lesions, which have been only unilateral, would thus have a
more devastating effect on one direction of horizontal movements
than on vertical movements.

A large variety of more "loosely coupled" burst neurons are
also found in the PRF. The behavior of these cells would seem to
place them at more central levels from the type just previously
described.

Henn and Cohen (1976) have described two classes of burst cells
which fit in this latter group: One type is correlated in burst
duration with the vector amplitude (and hence duration) of the eye
movement independent of the direction of the movement. For the
other type, average discharge rate of the burst is approximated by a
function, $F \cos \alpha$, where F is some maximum frequency for each unit
and α is the angle of the eye movement measured in a conventional
polar coordinate system from a reference direction of either
horizontal or a direction tilted 10-20 deg from the vertical. They
have suggested that the signals from these directional coding cells
could interact in another cell (one with a multiplicative response
property) with inputs from the amplitude coding cells. The hypothesized result would be a resolution of the amplitude vector coding
activity into components for the horizontal and vertical medium-lead
burst cells previously discussed.

This explanation has some difficulties, since for most oblique
movements the vertical and horizontal components are not of the same
temporal duration. Thus a multiplicative interaction of the two
classes of PRF burst cells described by Henn and Cohen (1976) would
not produce component bursts of the proper duration for the horizontal and vertical medium-lead burst cells. Burst duration as was
previously discussed, appears to be the critical variable required
by both horizontal and vertical pools of motoneurons. In any case,
units coding direction of movements represented 9% of the total
sample of PRF units recorded by Henn and Cohen (1976).

Another intersting type of burst cell, called long-lead
bursters, constituted a significant percentage (12-20%) of the cells
encountered in the PRF. These cells were grouped together because
they displayed a relatively long (20-200 msec) prelude of irregular
discharge which usually preceded a more intense burst just prior to
the saccade (Lushei and Fuchs, 1972; Keller, 1974). One example of
this type of cell is shown in Fig. 4. This oversimplified classification scheme tends to obscure the fact that this group of cells
contains a complex mixture of subtypes most of which burst for
saccades in all directions, some showed occasional bursts of activity
in the absence of any eye movement, and some display periods of low-
frequency tonic discharge unrelated to eye movements. A majority of
those burst units coding direction of eye movement as previously
described belonged to this class of units (Henn and Cohen, 1976).

     Although we cannot assign an exact functional role to this type
of unit at the present time, their pattern of activity suggests that
they are certainly not immediate supranuclear cells, but instead may
play a role in activating other PRF units in preparation for an
approaching saccade. Others in this same group might be involved in
a coordinating and informational role with other motor and sensory
systems.

Pause Units. Units that paused for saccades constituted about 10%
of the PRF units reported by Keller (1974) and 14% of those reported
by Henn and Cohen (1976). The majority of these units paused for
saccades in all directions. One example is shown in Fig. 5. The
duration of the pause was about the same as the duration of the

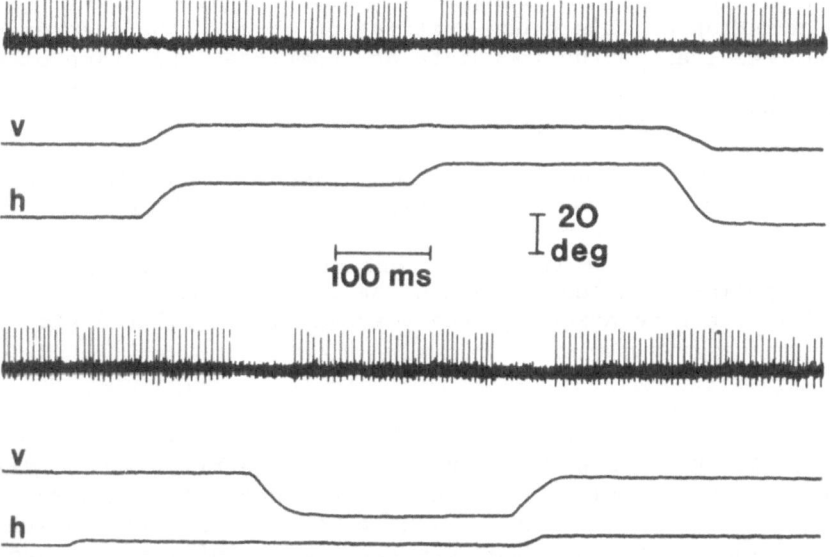

FIGURE 5. Activity of an omnidirectional pause unit during a se-
    quence of saccadic eye movements. In both sets of records
    upper trace is unit discharge, middle trace is vertical eye
    position, and lower trace is horizontal eye position.

movement, i.e., the duration of the larger component, either
vertical or horizontal. Thus this type of cell does not seem a
likely candidate for direct projection to the motoneuron pools.
Instead it has been suggested (Keller, 1974) that this group of
cells might powerfully inhibit the group of medium-lead burst
neurons. Since we hypothesize that this latter group projects
directly to oculomotor neurons, such a system would require that
medium-lead burst neurons never fire except when an eye movement
was commanded by a higher center. Spurious noise in this group of
cells would lead directly to small fixation changes which would be
intolerable for the visual system. The pause cells would prevent
this situation by their steady, high-frequency (100-200 spikes/sec)
tonic discharge which would be inhibitory on medium-lead burst
neurons. Brief cessation in this inhibitory discharge just prior
to and during the period of a desired saccade would allow the
discharge of a burst by the burst type cells.

This hypothesis is supported by the results obtained from
microstimulations in the vicinity of the pause units. While the
various types of burst units were found to be scattered throughout
the PRF, the location of most pause units was found to be more
discrete (Keller, 1974). There is a sharply defined concentration
of such neurons in a slender column running longitudinally along
the midline of the brain stem (Fig. 6A). The highest concentration
of these units was found in the midline in frontal planes at the
level of the ventrally coursing rootlets of the VIth nerve.
Microstimulation of this pause unit region through the recording
electrode resulted in the immediate and complete inhibition of all
saccadic eye movements for the duration of the stimulus train
(Keller, 1974) as shown in Fig. 6B.

Tonic Units. Evidence has been accumulating that the anatomic
areas immediately surrounding the abducens nucleus including
portions of the medullary and pontine reticular formation, the
most rostral part of the vestibular nucleus complex, and the prepositus hypoglossi nucleus, contain the cells (tonic units)
involved in the generation of steady eye-position related signals

FIGURE 6. A: Brain stem section cut in the vertical stereotaxic
    plane just rostral to the abducens nucleus. Arrow shows
    midline position of a small lesion at the recording location
    of a pause unit. B: Complete suppression of saccadic eye
    movements by electrical microstimulation at the pause unit
    recording site shown in A. Upper trace is vertical eye
    position,, middle trace is horizontal eye position, lower
    trace is the stimulus envelope. Time calibration in msec.

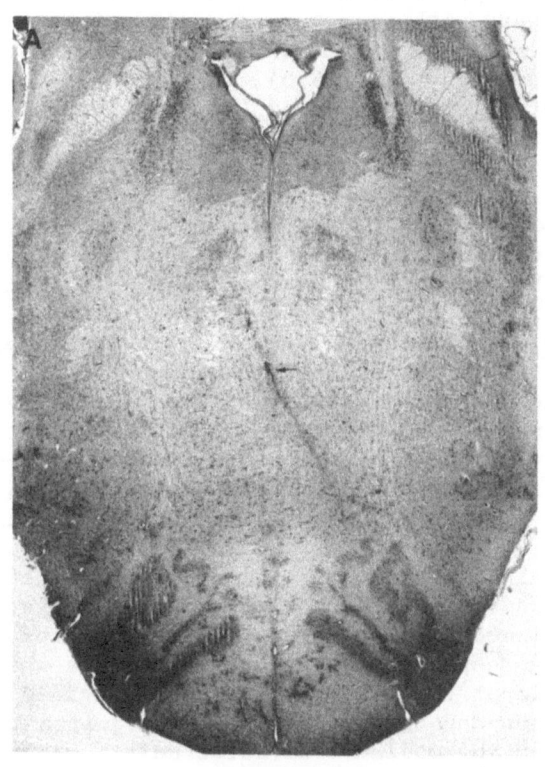

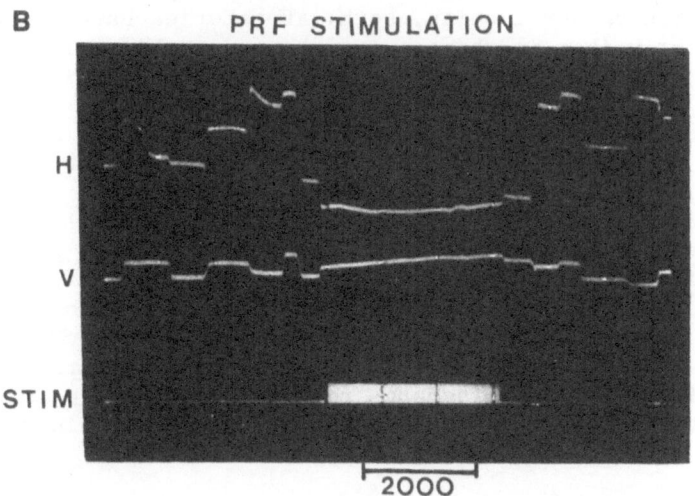

required by motoneurons during fixation (Luschei and Fuchs, 1972;
Keller, 1974; Miles, 1974; Baker et al., 1975; Keller and Daniels,
1975; Henn and Cohen, 1976; see also Baker, this conference).
Another commonly recorded type of neuron within all of these areas
is the burst-tonic type (Luschei and Fuchs, 1972). This distributed
anatomical structure with an apparent similar functional role may
also include interneurons within the anatomically defined abducens
nucleus (Baker and Highstein, 1975). A term used to define this
functional structure and which seems to be gaining general acceptance
is the oculomotor system integrator (Robinson, 1971).

     The concept of assigning a similar functional role to these
different anatomical areas is based on the similarity of the
response of tonic and burst-tonic neurons recorded in each area.
Thus far it has been possible only to judge this similarity on the
basis of a superficial comparison of the published responses
recorded in each of these areas. What is now required in order to
determine if all these areas share in the operation of the neural
integrator or whether there exist real differences in their contribution to the function of this key element in the oculomotor
system, is a careful quantitative and comparative study of the
parameters describing the discharge behavior and its relation to
eye movement for a large number of these units in each area.

     Beyond defining the anatomic locations of the oculomotor
integrator, one would like to be able to explain its operation in
terms of neuronal mechanisms. A start in this direction has been
made by recording responses in the PRF of neurons which could
function as the input to the integrator for saccadic eye movements
(Keller, 1974; Henn and Cohen, 1976). The required response seems
to be furnished by the medium-lead burst unit (unit coding change
of position of Henn and Cohen, 1976). As was previously discussed
in the section on burst units, both laboratories have found that
the number of spikes in these units' bursts is linearly related to
the size of the component of eye movement in the on-direction of
the unit. Even a single cell of this type discharges a remarkably
accurate code of the change in eye position occurring during its
burst. It was usually possible to determine within one degree the
size of the horizontal component of eye movement from counting the
number of discharges occurring in the burst of a single medium-
lead burster during the movement. Any simple type of population
averaging on these units would provide a signal of sufficient
accuracy to code the change of eye position. Thus, conceptually
the neural integrator could function as a network which counts the
number of spikes present in its input (medium-lead burster terminals)
and maintains an output discharge rate proportional to this input.
This output essentially describes the behavior of tonic cells.

One ramification of this hypothesis would be that collaterals of the same group of medium-lead burst cells could supply the signal to be integrated for the step, and hence eventual fixation position, and also directly to motoneurons, the pulse to provide the high-velocity saccadic movement. It's clear from studies of ocular mechanics that the pulse and step portions of the combined oculo-motor neuron control signal are not independent variables. Each duration and intensity of pulse corresponds to a specific step (fixation change). By coding both these changes in a single pool of cells the central nervous system could vastly simplify the necessity for coordination of these components.

ELECTROPHYSIOLOGICAL AND ANATOMICAL TRACING OF PRF CONNECTIONS

The results obtained from electrophysiological experiments conducted on the PRF confirm some of the impressions formed from the single-unit recording studies previously mentioned. Monosynaptic PSPs were elicited in identified oculomotor and abducens nucleus motoneurons following electrical stimulation of the PRF in cat (Highstein et al., 1974; Kaneko et al., 1975; Highstein, 1976). The pattern of these projections to the oculomotor nucleus included EPSPs to all the subgroups of motoneurons suggesting a role for the PRF in vertical eye movements similar to the impression gained from the single-unit work. The pattern of projections to the oculomotor nucleus included EPSPs to the ipsilateral and IPSPs to the contra-lateral motoneurons. The majority of the EPSPs did not occlude with incoming vestibular signals either from the MLF (oculomotor neurons) or directly from the VN (abducens neurons) demonstrating a separate PRF input pathway in addition to the well-known vestibulo-ocular pathways.

In these same studies cells in the PRF which project directly to the IIIrd and VIth nuclei were identified by intracellular recordings of their antidromic action potentials subsequent to stimulation in the region of the IIIrd and VIth nuclei.

Results which are in partial confirmation of these electrophy-siological studies have been obtained from histologic tracing techniques. The injection of the retrograde tracer, horseradish peroxidase, into the region of the IIIrd nucleus and the VIth nucleus has revealed PRF inputs to only the latter nucleus in cat (Graybiel and Hartwieg, 1974; Kaneko et al., 1975) and in monkey (Graybiel, 1975). Similar findings have resulted from the appli-cation of anterograde autoradiographic techniques, namely confirmation of the presence of cell bodies in the PRF projecting directly to the vicinity of the VIth nucleus, but not the IIIrd nucleus (Graybiel and Hartwieg, 1974; Büttner-Ennever and Henn, 1976).

These anatomic findings coupled with the observation that
fibers in the MLF, which are presumedly projecting directly to
motoneurons, already possess a fully assembled (burst-tonic) oculomotor neuron control signal, raise some serious doubts about the
role of the direct PRF oculomotor nucleus neuron projection. It
seems entirely possible that one output of the PRF, which on the
basis of the single-unit recording studies in alert animals is
thought to consist of axons of the medium-lead burst cells, projects
directly to abducens motoneurons and to burst-tonic neurons in the
previously discussed parabducens complex. This projection would
provide directly to abducens motoneurons, and indirectly via one
additional synapse and the MLF to medial rectus motoneurons, the
source of their burst (pulse) signal. In this hypothesis the same
neurons also project directly to tonic cells in the parabducens
complex for integration to the step signal and reprojection in
parallel to burst-tonic cells and abducens motoneurons.

INPUTS FROM THE SUPERIOR COLLICULUS TO THE PRF

Attention is now focused on a portion of the results from a new
study which sheds some additional light on the organization of the
PRF and its role in the control of eye movements. In recent investigation we (Raybourn and Keller, unpublished results) system-
atically stimulated the superior colliculus (SC) with focal electrical stimulation whilst simultaneously recording in turn from a
large sample of each of the types of PRF units previously discussed.
Since the SC is widely believed to be a higher level neural structure
integrating visual-oculomotor behavior, we hoped to clarify some of
the relations among the various types of PRF cells by careful
observation of the neural events occurring in the PRF following the
stimulations of the SC with shocks both above and below the threshold
for generating eye movements.

In addition to the various types of eye movement-related (EMR)
neurons previously reported in the PRF, we also recorded from a
large number of non-eye movement-related (NEMR) cells in this
study. A higher percentage of NEMR cells could be activated by SC
stimulation than EMR types, but at significantly longer latencies.
Among the EMR cells the inputs from SC were very specific and
consistent. Each long-lead burst neuron in the PRF received short-
latency (mono- to disynaptic) input from all regions of the
colliculus. Reverberatory firing behavior was elicited in these
cells by single-pulse collicular stimulations which raises the
possibility of the temporal encoding mechanisms being contained
within the ensemble activity of these neurons. Long-lead burst
neurons could be consistently activated by SC stimulation at current
levels well below those required to produce saccadic eye movements.

Juxtathreshold (for eye movements) SC stimulation also resulted in a mono- to disynaptic excitation-inhibition sequence in pauser cells in the PRF. The duration of pauser cell inhibition (or disfacilitation) was graded with collicular stimulation intensities.

Collicular input to eye position dependent PRF neurons (tonic, burst-tonic) was less extensive and at longer synaptic latencies than to saccadic-related neurons. Medium-lead burster units and abducens motoneurons were not synaptically driven by collicular stimulation in this alert preparation. In addition, tonic and burst-tonic cells were only activated at stimulation levels which consistently evoked saccadic eye movements.

These data support the hypothesis that long-lead burst neurons are the PRF cell type forming the interface between higher visual centers like the SC and the more immediate supranuclear elements -- the medium-lead burst type. The former type begins to discharge well before the onset of saccadic movements at about the time that movement related cells in the intermediate and deep layer of the colliculus become active (see Sparks, this symposium). In contrast to collicular eye movement related cells, these PRF burst cells do not appear to have any movement field (spatial) organization. Thus the transformation from spatial coding present in the SC appears to be partially transformed into the temporal coding (pulse duration) required by motoneurons at the level of long-lead burst neurons. Therefore we suggest that this cell type plays a pivotal role in PRF saccadic organization.

ACKNOWLEDGEMENTS

Research sponsored by the National Institutes of Health Grant EY 00955-05.

REFERENCES

1. Baker, R. and Berthoz, A. Organization of vestibular nystagmus
    in oblique oculomotor system. *J. Neurophysiol.* 37:195-217,
    1974.

2. Baker, R. Gresty, M. and Berthoz, A. Neuronal activity in the
    prepositus hypoglossi nucleus correlated with vertical and
    horizontal eye movement in the cat. *Brain Res.* 101:366-371,
    1975.

3. Baker, R. and Highstein, S. M. Physiological identification
    of interneurons and motoneurons in the abducens nucleus.
    Brain Res. 91:292-298, 1975.

4. Barmack, N.H. Saccadic discharges evoked by intracellular
    stimulation of extraocular motoneurons. *J. Neurophysiol.*
    37:395-412, 1974.

5. Büttner-Ennever, J. A. and Henn, V. An autoradiographic study
    of the pathways from the pontine reticular formation involved
    in horizontal eye movements. *Brain Res.* 108:155-164, 1976.

6. Cohen, R. and Henn, V. Unit activity in the pontine reticular
    formation associated with eye movements. *Brain Res.*
    46:403-410, 1972a.

7. Cohen, B. and Henn, V. The origin of the quick phases of
    nystagmus in the horizontal plane. In: *Cerebral Control of
    Eye Movements and Motion Perception.* Dichgans, J. and Bizzi,
    E. (eds). *Biblo. Ophthal.,* 82:36-55, Karger: Basel, 1972b.

8. Cohen, B., Komatsuzaki, A. and Bender, M. B. Electrooculographic
    syndrome in monkeys after pontine reticular formation lesions.
    Arch. Neurol. Chicago 18:78-92, 1968.

9. Davis-King, W. M., Lisberger, S. G., Fuchs, A. F., and Evinger,
    L. C. Activity of simian MLF fibers related to eye movement
    and adequate vestibular stimulation. *Neurosci. Abstr.* 1:185,
    1975.

10. Fuchs, A. F. and Kimm, J. Unit activity in vestibular nucleus
    of the alert monkey during horizontal angular acceleration
    and eye movement. *J. Neurophysiol.* 38:1140-1161, 1975.

11. Graybiel, A. M. Anatomical pathways in the brain stem
    oculomotor system. In: *Eye Movements and Motion Perception,*
    Ninth Symp. Center Visual Science, Rochester, N. Y., 1975.

12. Graybiel, A. M. and Hartwieg, E. A. Some afferent connections of the oculomotor complex in the cat: an experimental study with tracer techniques. *Brain Res*. 81:543–551, 1974.

13. Henn, V. and Cohen, B. Quantitative analysis of activity in eye muscle motoneurons during saccadic eye movement and positions of fixation. *J. Neurophysiol*. 36:115–126, 1973.

14. Henn, V. and Cohen, B. Coding of information about rapid eye movements in the pontine reticular formation of alert monkeys'. *Brain Res*. 108:307–325, 1976.

15. Highstein, S. M., and Cohen, B. and Matsunami, K. Monosynaptic projections from the pontine reticular formation to the IIIrd nucleus in the cat. *Brain Res*. 75:340–344, 1974.

16. Kaneko, C. R. S., Steinacker, A., Cohen, B., Maciewicz, R. and Highstein, S. M. Synaptic linkage of the reticuloocular pathway in the cat. *Neurosci. Abstr*. 1:349, 1975.

17. Keller, E. L. Participation of medial pontine reticular formation associated with eye movements. *J. Neurophysiol*. 37: 316–332, 1974.

18. Keller, E. L. and Daniels, P. D. Oculomotor related interaction of vestibular and visual stimulation in vestibular nucleus cells in alert monkey. *Exptl. Neurol*. 46:187–198, 1975.

19. Keller, E. L. and Robinson, D. A. Absence of a stretch reflex in extraocular muscles of the monkey. *J. Neurophysiol*. 34:908–919, 1971.

20. Luschei, E. S. and Fuchs, A. F. Activity of brain stem neurons during eye movements of alert monkeys. *J. Neurophysiol*. 35:455–461, 1972.

21. Maeda, M., Shimazu, H., and Shinoda, Y. Nature of synaptic events in cat abducens motoneurons at slow and quick phase of vestibular nystagmus. *J. Neurophysiol*. 35:279–296, 1972.

22. Miles, F. A. Single unit firing patterns in the vestibular nuclei related to voluntary eye movements and passive body rotation in conscious monkeys. *Brain Res*. 71:215–224, 1974.

23. Olszewski, J. The cytoarchitecture of the human reticular formation. In: *Brain Mechanisms and Consciousness*. ed. Adrian, E. D., Bremer, F. and Jasper, M.H. pp. 54–80, Oxford: Blackwell, 1954.

24. Pola, J. MLF fiber activity in monkey during visually elicited and vestibular eye movement. *Neurosci. Abstr.* 1:377.

25. Robinson, D. A. Oculomotor unit behavior in the monkey. *J. Neurophysiol.* 33:393-404, 1970.

26. Robinson, D. A. Models of oculomotor neural organization. In: *The Control of Eye Movements.* ed. Bach-y-Rita, P. and Collins, C.C., pp. 519-538, New York:Academic, 1971.

27. Robinson, D. A. and Keller, E. L. The behavior of eye movement motoneurons in the later monkey. In *Cerebral Control of Eye Movements and Motion Perception.*, *Bibl. Ophthal.* 82:36-55, Basel:Karger.

28. Sasaki, K. Electrophysiological studies on oculomotor neurons of the cat. *Jap. J. Physiol.* 13:287-302, 1963.

29. Sparks, D. L. and Travis, R. F. Firing patterns of reticular formation neurons during horizontal eye movements. *Brain Res.* 33:477-481, 1971.

ABDUCENS TO MEDIAL RECTUS PATHWAY IN THE MLF: A POSSIBLE

CELLULAR BASIS FOR THE SYNDROME OF INTERNUCLEAR OPHTHALMOPLEGIA

Stephen M. Highstein
Department of Neuroscience
Division of Cellular Neurobiology
Albert Einstein College of Medicine
Bronx, New York

The neurological syndrome of internuclear ophthalmoplegia consists of defects in horizontal and vertical eye movements: a prominent feature is the loss of conjugate horizontal gaze (Bender & Weinstein, 1944; Cogan, 1948; Cogan et al., 1960; Christoff et al., 1960; Carpenter & McMasters, 1963; Carpenter & Strominger, 1965; Cohen, 1971). Horizontal gaze deficits are caused by an apparent palsy of the medial rectus extraocular muscle which is manifested as a weakness of medially directed gaze in the affected eye. With interruption of/or damage to the medial longitudinal fasciculus (MLF) on one side, the ipsilateral eye is abducted at rest and does not cross into the nasal or medial field of gaze except during convergence movements. Medially directed saccades in the affected eye are slowed (Evinger et al., in press) and neither vestibular, visual nor voluntarily induced eye movement can cause the eye to deviate into the medial hemifield (Evinger et al., in press; Cohen, 1971). It is noted that the adductive paresis is also present during electrical stimulation of the pontine reticular formation, a powerful stimulus which usually produces ipsilaterally directed conjugate horizontal eye movement (Cohen, 1974). The profound nature of this adductive paresis implies the necessity of an intact MLF for the production of all conjugate horizontal eye movements (Cohen, 1971; Cohen, 1974).

By contrast, in the intact animal (monkey or cat, and by inference man) unilateral electrical stimulation of the intact MLF produces an ipsilateral medial rectus muscle activation and adduction of the ipsilateral eye (Bender & Weinstein, 1944; Cohen, 1971). Thus the apparent deficits in eye movement after damage to the MLF are presumably due to a decrease in the ascending tonic excitation

to the medial rectus motoneurons causing ocular malposition at
rest, and the interruption of the ascending synchronized excitatory
command signals which produce medially directed eye movements.
Fig. 1B is a photograph of a monkey with a documented lesion in
the right MLF between the oculomotor and abducens nuclei. Note
that there is a paresis of right ocular adduction on attempted
left lateral gaze. This monkey demonstrated typical internuclear
ophthalmoplegia; the lesion in the MLF was verified histologically
(Fig. 1A).

    Although the importance of the MLF in organizing conjugate
horizontal gaze has never been doubted, it has previously been
assumed that interruption of ascending secondary vestibular fibers
in the MLF or fibers from the reticular formation entering the MLF
to ascend to the medial rectus motoneurons is causative in producing
internuclear ophthalmoplegia. It will be shown below that this is
probably not the case. Although many fibers originating in the
vestibular nuclei have been shown to ascend in the MLF (Tarlov,
1970; Cohen, 1971; Gacek, 1971; Highstein et al., 1971; Highstein,
1973), a specific group of secondary vestibular fibers which
terminate upon medial rectus motoneurons has not been demonstrated.
The existence of fibers from the reticular formation entering into
the MLF and terminating upon medial rectus motoneurons has also
been postulated for many years but again has not been verified
experimentally.

    A recent morphological study employing the retrograde tracer
horseradish peroxidase injected into the oculomotor nucleus suggests
that there are neurones within the abducens nucleus which are not
motoneurons and which project (presumably via the MLF) to the
contralateral oculomotor complex (Graybiel et al., 1974). These
morphological results are at variance with those of Warwick (1964)
who suggested that all cells lying within the abducens nucleus are
motoneurons. The identification of motoneurons, and non-motoneurons
within the abducens nuclear complex has also recently been explored
electrophysiologically (Baker and Highstein, 1975). Fig. 2 diagrams
the experimental paradigm employed. Anesthetized, paralyzed, and
artificially respired cats were mounted in a stereotaxic apparatus.
Both abducens nerves to the lateral rectus muscles were isolated
and stimulated in the orbits. In addition, electrodes were implanted
in both labyrinths and a stimulating electrode was placed in the
MLF just posterior to the oculomotor nucleus. The cerebellum was
removed and microelectrodes were introduced into the region of the
abducens nucleus in order to record from motoneurons and possibly
other cells within the nucleus. Abducens motoneurons (AbdMns)
were identified by their antidromic responses to stimulation of
the abducens nerve in the orbit (Fig. 3 Abd, Baker et al., 1969).
In no case was an abducens motoneuron thus identified antidromically
activated by stimulation within the MLF. This is strong presumptive

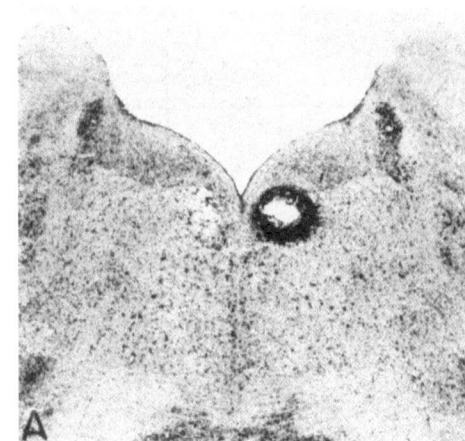 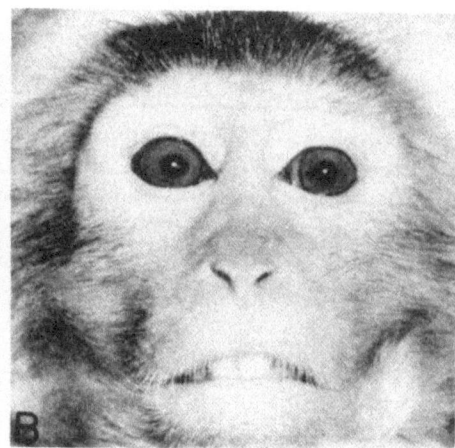

FIGURE 1. Eye movement deficit secondary to MLF lesion.

A. A discrete lesion in the right MLF rostral to the
abducens nucleus. Cresyl violet stain.

B. Photograph of lesioned animal showing paresis of right
ocular adduction on attempted left lateral gaze.

Reproduced from text – Fig. 9, p. 85 in The Control of
Eye Movements (Eds.) P. Bach-y-Rita, C. C. Collins and J. E.
Hyde, NY: Academic Press, 1971 with the permission of Prof.
M. B. Carpenter.

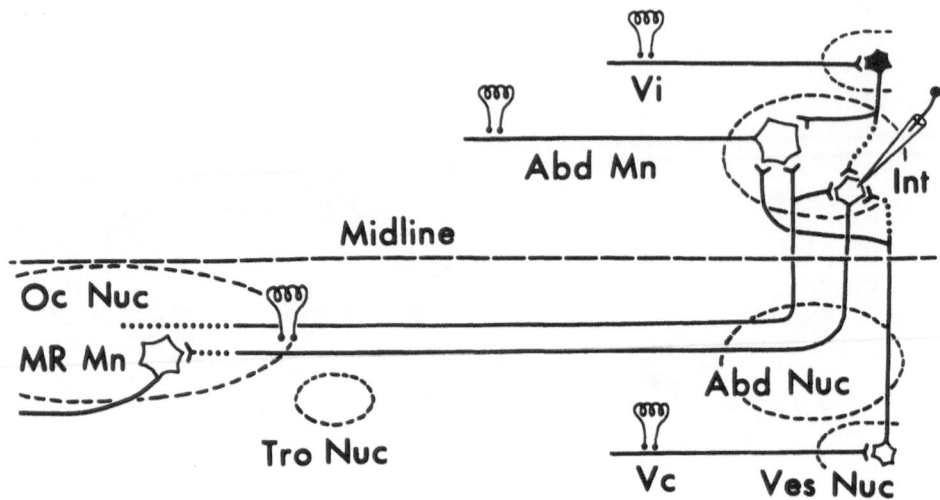

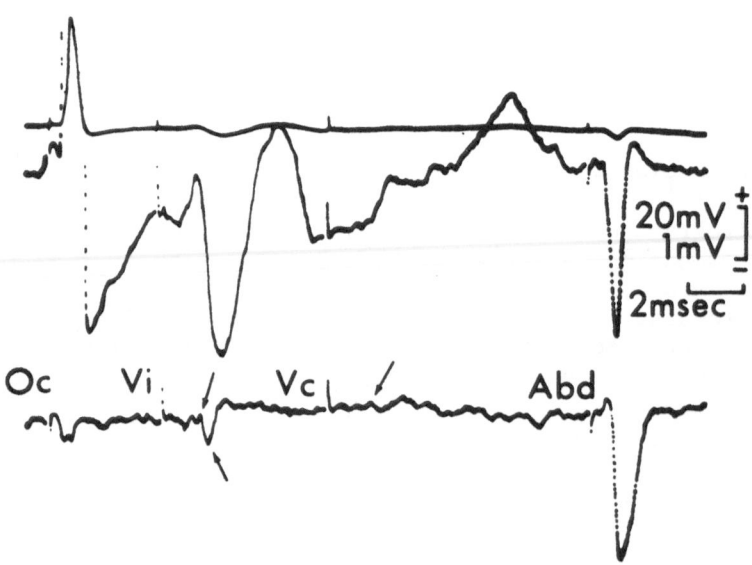

FIGURE 2. Schematic diagram of the experimental paradigm with
    intracellular anti- and orthodromic activity recorded from an
    abducens internuclear neuron identified within the abducens
    nucleus. Diagram, intracellular recordings were obtained from
    internuclear neurons (Int) in the abducens nucleus following
    stimulation of the ipsilateral (Vi) or contralateral (Vc)
    vestibular nerve, oculomotor (Oc) and abducens nerve. The
    dotted lines indicate the pathways likely to mediate the
    anti- and orthodromic connections suggested in this study.
    In the records below, the upper two traces are intracellular
    and the lower (marked one) is the extracellular response.
    The upper intracellular record is a high gain AC coupled trace
    and the middle a low gain DC coupled record. Sequential Oc
    (3x threshold), Vi (2x threshold), Vc (2x threshold) and Abd
    (5x threshold) stimulation. The arrows indicate latency for
    orthodromic synaptic responses. Note the absence of antidromic
    activation of the neuron in response to Abd stimulation.

        Modified from Baker and Highstein, 1975.

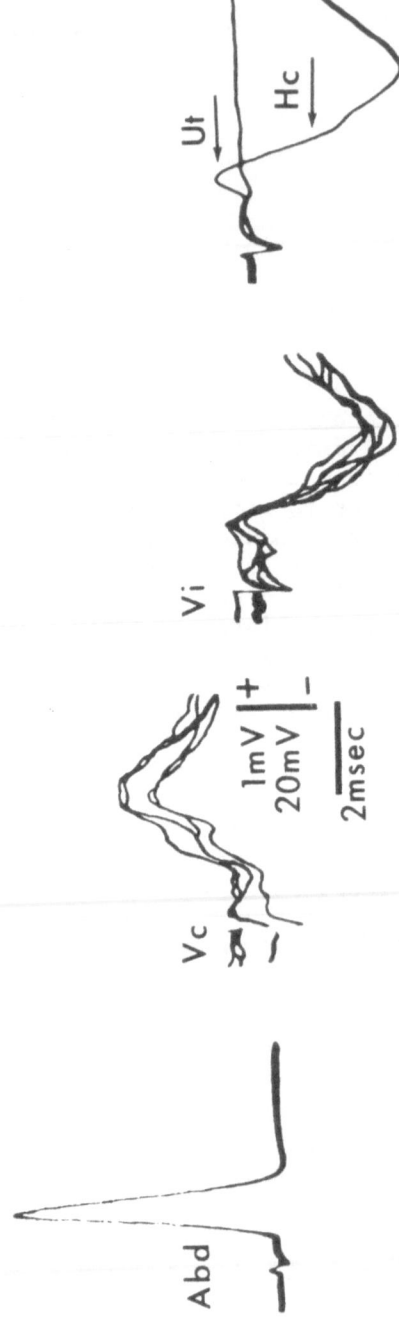

FIGURE 3. Postsynaptic potential recorded from abducens motoneurons after gross stimulation of the ipsilateral and contralateral VIIIth nerve.

Intracellular recordings from abducens motoneurons in response to stimulation of the VIth nerve (Abd), the contralateral VIIIth nerve (Vc), the ipsilateral VIIIth nerve (Vi) and superposition of intra- and extracellular response following ipsilateral VIIIth nerve stimulation (16 averaged traces). Schwindt et al., demonstrated that the disynaptic EPSP arises from stimulation of the ipsilateral utricular nerve (UT), while the IPSP arises from ipsilateral horizontal canal stimulation (Hc).

Modified from Schwindt et al., 1973 with the permission of Prof. W. Precht.

evidence that AbdMns do not have axon collaterals which ascend in
the MLF. Another class of neurone was rather less frequently
impaled in the abducens nucleus. These cells did respond to
stimulation of the MLF with the generation of antidromic action
potentials as is illustrated in Fig. 2, but did not respond with
synaptic or antidromic potentials to stimulation of the abducens
nerve within the orbit. Thus these cells lying within the cellular
confines of the abducens nucleus are not AbdMns. We have tentatively
named them internuclear neurons of the abducens nucleus (AbIns).
The profile of synaptic potentials induced in AbIns by stimulation
of the ipsilateral and contralateral labyrinths is also illustrated
in Fig. 2. Stimulation of the ipsilateral labyrinth (Vi) produces
a disynaptic EPSP followed by an IPSP while stimulation of the
contralateral labyrinth (Vc) produces a disynaptic EPSP. A comparison
of these labyrinthine evoked synaptic potentials in AbIns to those
in AbdMns (Richter and Precht, 1968; Baker et al., 1969; Schwint
et al., 1973) indicates that AbIns receive the exact same profile
of synaptic excitation and inhibition from the labyrinths as do
the AbdMns (Fig. 3). These synaptic potentials in AbMns presumably
underlie the contraction and relaxation of the lateral rectus eye
muscles which participate in the compensatory eye movements produced
by adequate labyrinthine stimulation. Thus the synaptic drive on
the AbIns from the vestibular labyrinth is identical to that upon
abducens motoneurons. This suggests that these cells probably
respond just in phase with abducens motoneurons during adequate
labyrinthine stimulation.

      In addition the nuclei of the pontine reticular formation,
the Nucleus reticularis pontis oralis (N. r. p. o.) and caudalis
(N. r. p. c.) have long been known to be intimately involved in
horizontal gaze mechanisms (Lorente de No, 1928; Cohen et al.,
1968; Cohen, 1971; Cohen and Henn, 1972a; Cohen and Komatsuzaki,
1972b; Cohen, 1974; Keller, 1974; Henn and Cohen, 1976; Highstein
et al., 1976). Stimulation in the region of these nuclei produces
ipsilateral horizontal eye movements (Cohen et al., 1972a) while
ablation leads to a prolonged paralysis of conjugate horizontal
eye movements in the ipsilateral hemifield of gaze (Cohen et al.,
1968). Employing an acute electrophysiological paradigm similar
to that in Fig. 3, it has been demonstrated that stimulation of
the region of the N. r. p. c. and N. r. p. o. evokes EPSPs
monosynaptically in ipsilateral AbIns (Fig. 4C) and AbdMns (Highstein
et al., 1976). This projection has been confirmed morphologically
by orthograde transport of labeled amino acids from the N. r. p.
c. and N. r. p. o. region to the abducens nucleus (Buttner-Enniver
and Henn, 1976; Graybiel, submitted for publication). Stimulation
of the contralateral N.r.p.c. and N.r.p.o. evokes predominantly
disynaptic IPSPs in the AbIns (Fig. 4B) and AbdMns. These IPSPs
are apparently transmitted through the inhibitory secondary
vestibular interneurons to AbdMns and AbIns (Highstein et al.,
1976).

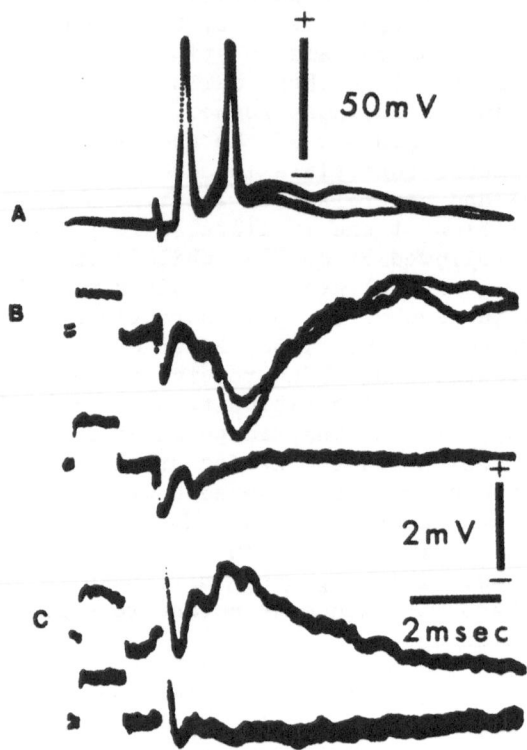

FIGURE 4. Postsynaptic potentials recorded from an internuclear neuron of the abducens nucleus.

A. Intracellular records from an adbucens internuclear neuron in response to stimulation of the MLF in the region of the IIIrd nucleus.

B. Stimulation of the contralateral Nucleus reticularis pontis caudalis and pontis oralis.

C. Stimulation of the ipsilateral N.r.p.c. and p.o. Upper records in B, C are intracellular and lower are extracellular controls.

Modified from Highstein et al., 1976.

In order to determine the sites of termination of the AbIns, morphologicical studies employing the orthograde transport of radioactive amino acids have been undertaken. When H^3-proline is injected into the abducens nucleus, axon terminals labeled with radioactive material can be seen in the IIIrd nucleus (Graybiel and Hartwieg, 1974). This indicates that there are cells within the vicinity of the abducens nucleus which take up the amino acids, incorporate them into proteins, and transport these proteins upstream to their axon terminals. These labeled axon terminals are localized to the subdivision of the contralateral oculomotor nuclear complex which contains the motoneurons innervating the medial rectus extraocular muscle. Because the labyrinthine and reticular inputs to the AbIns are in phase with those in abducens motoneurons (Figs 3,4) it was postulated that the AbIns would terminate with excitation upon contralateral medial rectus moto-neurons (Baker and Highstein, 1975) and thus would regulate conjugate horizontal gaze in the two eyes. In order to investigate this projection electrophysiologically the paradigm illustrated in Fig. 5 was undertaken. Similar to Fig. 2, both labyrinths were stimulated. However, in this case the medial rectus nerve in the orbit was placed on stimulating electrodes to antidromically identify medial rectus motoneurons. In addition a stimulating electrode was placed within the contralateral abducens nucleus; both MLFs were also stimulated. When the recording microelectrode was placed in the dorsolateral subdivision of the oculomotor nuclear complex a large antidromic field potential was produced by stimu-lation of the medial rectus nerve (Fig. 5, lower right). Ipsilateral labyrinthine stimulation produced a sharp transient field potential followed by a slight negativity while contralateral abducens nucleus stimulation produced a remarkable field potential consisting of an early biphasic sharp transient followed by a later negativity (Fig. 5, lower trace, middle). The early transient presumably represents the incoming volley of the axons of the AbIns while the later negativity indicates postsynaptic EPSPs and activation of medial rectus motoneurones. Intracellular recording demonstrates that stimulation of the contralateral abducens nucleus produces large EPSPs in identified medial rectus motoneurons (Fig. 6 Highstein and Baker, in preparation). Latency to onset of these EPSPs following contralateral abducens nucleus stimulation averaged 0.5 msec, well within the monosynaptic range. These EPSPs were often suprathreshold for spike initiation (lower traces, Fig. 6). Fig. 7 compares the amplitudes of the EPSPs produced from stimulation of the abducens nucleus with those produced from stimulation of the ipsilateral labyrinth (Vi). The abducens evoked EPSPs are similar in amplitude to those produced by Vi stimulation (Fig. 7, B) and in addition they increase and decrease their amplitude with the passage of hyper and depolarizing currents through the micro-electrode in parallel with the Vi evoked EPSPs (Fig. 7 A, and C). Reversal of the Abd and Vi induced EPSPs was at the same membrane

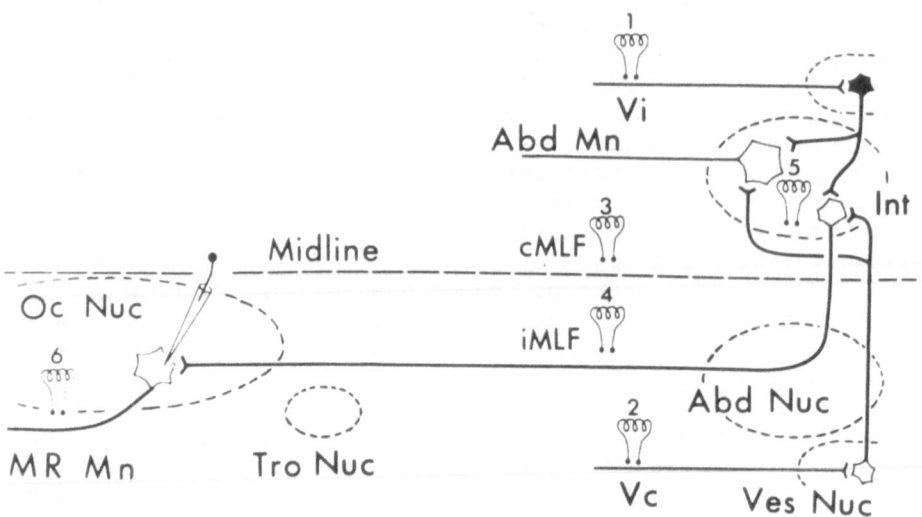

DORSOLATERAL MR SUBDIVISION

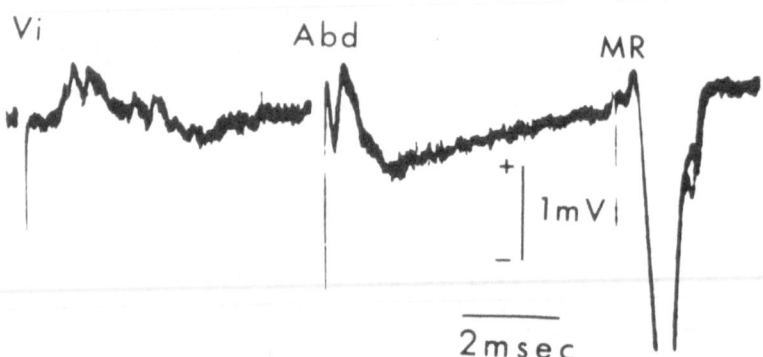

FIGURE 5. Schematic diagram of the experimental paradigm with extracellular field potentials recorded in the medial rectus subdivision of the oculomotor nucleus.

Diagram, intra- and extracellular recordings were obtained from the medial rectus subdivision of the oculomotor nucleus (OcNuc) following stimulation of the ipsilateral vestibular nerve (Vi), the abducens nucleus (AbdNuc) and the nerve to the medial rectus muscle. Vc is the contralateral vestibular nerve. MRMn is a medial rectus motoneuron and iMLF and cMLF are the ipsi- and contralateral MLFs respectively.

The extracellular records below were produced in response to stimulation of Vi, Abd, and the nerve to MR.

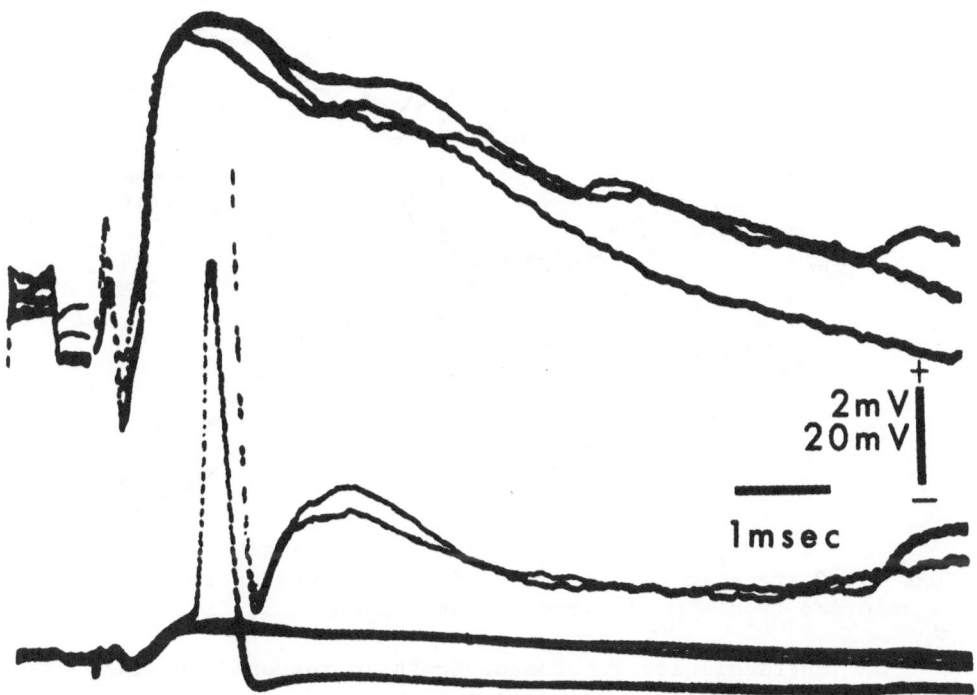

FIGURE 6. Postsynaptic potentials recorded from a medial rectus motoneuron.
   Intracellular EPSPs monosynaptically evoked in response to contralateral abducens nucleus stimulation. Upper traces are AC coupled; voltage calibration 2 mV. Lower traces are DC coupled; voltage calibration 20 mV.

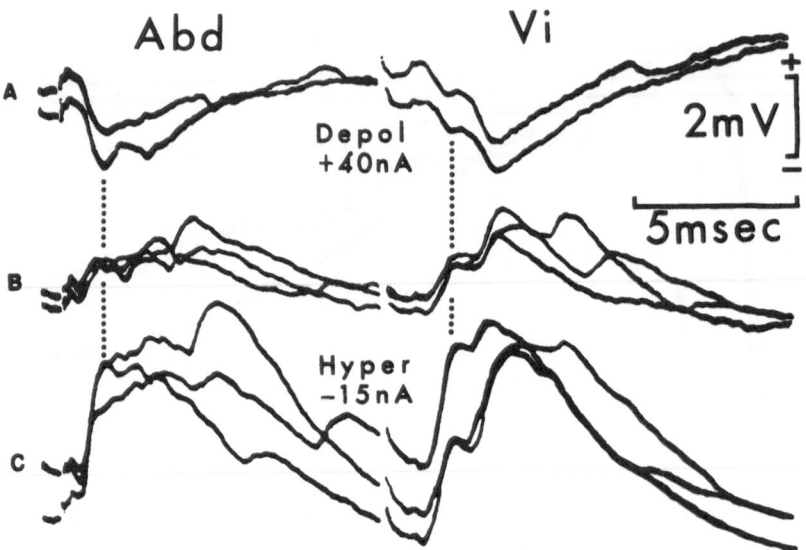

FIGURE 7. Current injection study of postsynaptic potentials recorded from a medial rectus motoneuron.

Intracellular records of EPSPs in response to stimulation of the contralateral abducens nucleus (Abd) and the ipsilateral vestibular nerve (Vi).

Control potentials are shown in B. In A. EPSPs have been reversed by the injection of +40 nA depolarizing currents through the recording microelectrode with a bridge circuit. In C, EPSP amplitudes have been increased by the passage −15 nA hyperpolarizing currents. Dotted lines indicate the initial peaks of the EPSPs.

potential implying similar synaptic sites and mechanisms for the
production of both of these potentials.

In order to investigate the uniqueness of the projection from
the contralateral abducens nucleus to the medial rectus motoneurons,
a series of chronic animals was prepared as illustrated in Fig. 8.
It was attempted in 4 animals to isolate the abducens nucleus from
structures which could possibly send axons or axon collaterals
through this nucleus. Knife cuts were placed as illustrated in
Fig. 8, and the animals allowed 4 days during which axons which
might be passing through or near the abducens nucleus could degen-
erate. The prepositus hypoglossi (8A) and the contralateral and
the ipsilateral vestibular nuclear complex (8A and C) as well as
the nucleus reticularis pontis oralis and caudalis (8B-D) were
surgically isolated from the abducens nucleus. Acute electrophysiology was performed four days after surgery on these cats
using the paradigm illustrated in Fig. 5. In all cases the
results were identical to unoperated controls, i.e. stimulation of
the contralateral abducens nucleus gave rise to monosynaptic EPSPs
in identified medial rectus motoneurons. We can therefore infer
the uniqueness of this projection which arises from the abducens
nucleus and ends upon medial rectus motoneurons (Highstein and
Baker, in preparation). That this projection is excitatory as
postulated indicates that the AbIns are ideally situated to organize
the action of the horizontal movers, i.e. the medial rectus
muscle of one eye and the lateral rectus of the other eye. Simultaneous activation of AbdMns and AbIns would therefore probably give
rise to conjugate horizontal eye movements. Interruption of the
axons of these AbIns within the MLF would result in a decrease of
tonic and phasic ascending excitation as well as possible absence
of disfacilitation travelling up the MLF to these medial rectus
motoneurons and thus could explain the syndrome of internuclear
ophthalmoplegia.

In additional experiments the pathways via which ascending
vestibular and reticular information reaches the IIIrd nucleus
have been carefully investigated (Baker and Highstein, in preparation).
No ascending vestibular or reticular projections to the medial
rectus motoneurons were found to lie within the MLF (Baker and
Highstein, in preparation; Highstein et al., 1974). This directly
implies that ascending information from the vestibular nuclei is
sent to the medial rectus subdivision of the oculomotor nuclear
complex by pathways other than the MLF. The prepositus hypoglossi
neurons do, however, ascend via the ipsilateral MLF to terminate
predominantly upon ipsilateral medial rectus motoneurons (Baker,
this volume; Baker et al., 1977). The relative importance and
function of these two ascending projections to medial rectus
neurons, i.e., prepositus, and AbIn, is currently being assessed.
With regard to this important question it is noted that a sagittal

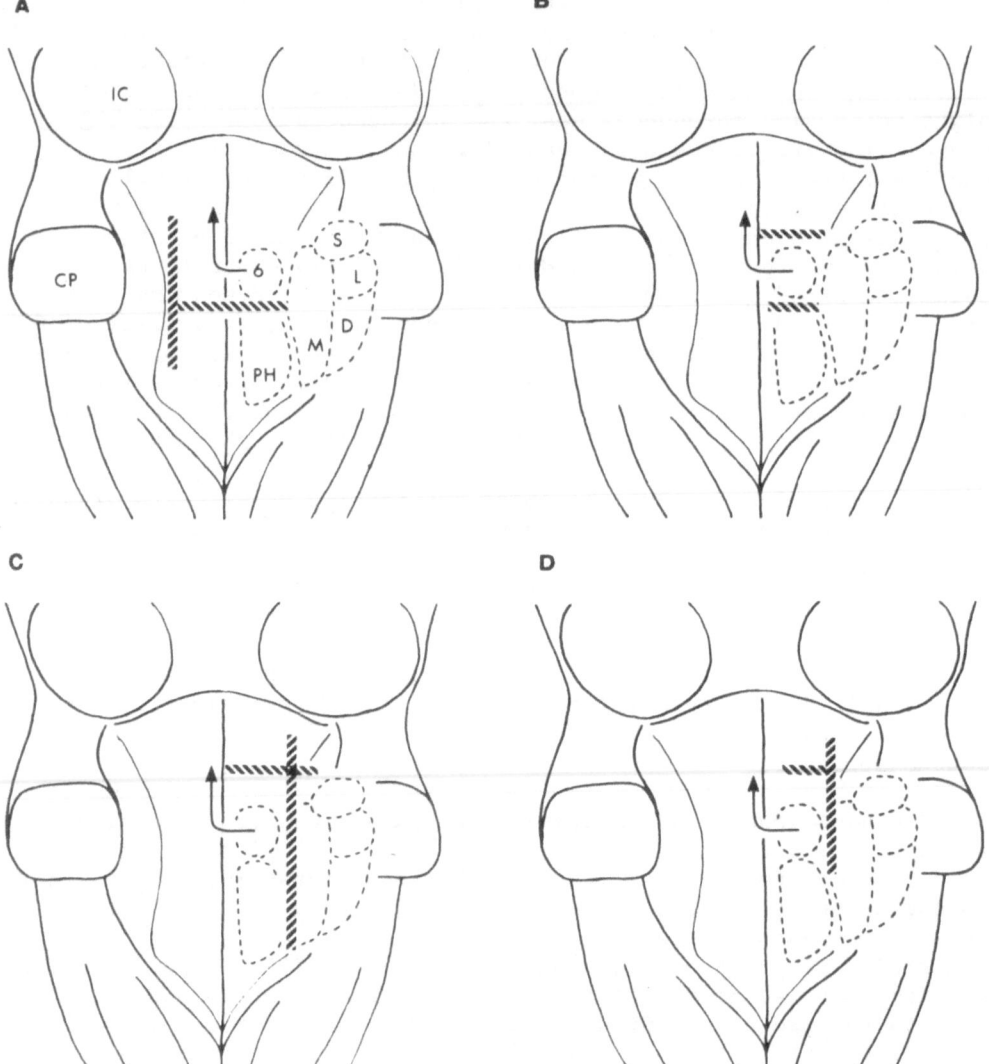

midline lesion between the abducens nuclei is sufficient to produce
bilateral internuclear ophthalmolplegia in both monkey (Cohen et
al., 1977) and cat (Baker, personal communication). A sagittal
knife cut at the level of the abducens nucleus will interrupt
the crossed internuclear pathway (but not the ipsilateral prepositus
projection) and thus it is probably the interruption of the axons
of the AbIns which accounts for internuclear ophthalmoplegia.

To date it appears that some ascending vestibular (Baker and
Highstein, in preparation), reticular (Highstein et al., 1976) and
possibly some of the prepositus hypoglossi signals (Maciewicz et
al., 1977) to medial rectus motoneurons are carried by the internuclear neurones which lie in the MLF. It may be postulated that
the predominant axons in the MLF related to horizontal eye movements
are the axons of the AbIns. These neurons are therefore probably
responsible for organizing the conjugate nature of horizontal
gaze; interruption of their axons may be sufficient to account for
the syndrome of internuclear ophthalmoplegia.

ACKNOWLEDGEMENTS

The author would like to express his gratitude to Ms. Ranjini Sekhar
for preparation of the manuscript. The research was supported by
NIH 5 KO4 EY00003-02, NIH 5 RO1 EY01670-02 and NS-07512.

FIGURE 8. Schematic representation of the lesions designed to
chronically isolate the abducens nucleus from surrounding
structures.

A-D. Lesions several mm deep (indicated by hatched lines)
were placed in the brainstem of 4 cats 4 days prior to the
acute recordings session.

A. The contralateral vestibular nuclear complex (S,L,
M,D, superior, lateral, medial and descending vestibular nuclei
respectively) and the ipsi- and contralateral nuclei prepositus
hypoglossi (PH) were isolated from the abducens nucleus (6).

B. The ipsilateral N.r.p.o. and p.c. was isolated from
the abducens nucleus. C,D. The ipsilateral N.r.p.c. and p.o.
and the ipsilateral vestibular nuclear complex were isolated
from the abducens nucleus. IC, inferior colliculus; CP,
cerebellar penduncle. The arrow indicates the presumed pathway of the axons of the AbIns.

REFERENCES

Baker, R.G., Mano, N., and Shimazu, H. Postsynaptic potentials in
    abducens motoneurons induced by vestibular stimulation.
    Brain Res., 15:577-580, 1969.

Baker, R. and Highstein, S.M. Physiological identification of
    interneurons and motoneurons in the abducens nucleus. *Brain
    Res.*, 91:292-298, 1975.

Baker, R., Delgado-Garcia, J. and Alley, K. Morphological and
    physiological demonstration that prepositus hypoglossi
    neurons terminate on medial rectus motoneurons. Abs. *Intn'l
    Cong. Physiol. Sci.*, in press, 1977.

Baker, R. and Highstein, S.M. The vestibular projection to medial
    rectus motoneurons. In preparation.

Baker, R. The Nucleus Prepositus Hypoglossi. This volume.

Baker, R. Personal communication.

Bender, M.B. and Weinstein, E.A. Effects of stimulation and
    lesion of the medial longitudinal fasiculus in the monkey.
    Arch. Neurol. Psychiat. (Chic.), 52:106-113, 1944.

Büttner-Ennever, J.A. and Henn, V. An autoradiographic study of
    the pathways from the pontine reticular formation involved in
    horizontal eye movements. *Brain Res.*, 108:155-164, 1976.

Carpenter, M.B. Central oculomotor pathways. In: *The Control of
    Eye Movements*, (Eds.) P. Bach-y-Rita and C.C. Collins, New
    York: Academic Press, 1971, pp. 67-104.

Carpenter, M.B. and McMasters, R.E. Disturbances of conjugate
    horizontal eye movement in the monkey. II. Physiological
    effects and anatomical degeneration resulting from lesions in
    the medial longitudinal fasiculus. *Arch. of Neurol.*, 8:347-
    368, 1963.

Carpenter, M.B. and Strominger, N.L. The medial longitudinal
    fasiculus and disturbances of conjugate horizontal eye movements
    in the monkey. *J. Comp. Neurol.*, 125:41-66, 1965.

Christoff, N., Anderson, P., Nathanson, M. and Bender, M.B.
    Problems in anatomic analysis of lesions of the medial longi-
    tudinal fasciculus. *Arch. Neurol. (Chic.)*, 2:293-304, 1960.

Cogan, D.G. Neurologic significance of lateral conjugate devia-
    tion of the eyes on forced closure of the lids. *Arch. Ophthal.*
    (Chic.), 39:37-42, 1948.

Cogan, D.G., Kubik, C.S., Smith, W.L. Unilateral internuclear
    ophthalmoplegia. Report of eight clinical cases with one
    postmortem study. *Arch. Ophthal. (Chic.)*, 44:783-796, 1960.

Cohen, B. Vestibulo-ocular relations. In: *The Control of Eye*
    Movements, (Eds.) P. Bach-y-Rita and C.C. Collins, New York:
    Academic Press, pp. 105-148, 1971.

Cohen, B. The Vestibulo-ocular reflex arc. In: *Handbook of*
    Sensory Physiology, Vol. 6, (Ed.) H.H. Kornhuber, Berlin:
    Springer Verlag, pp. 447-540, 1974.

Cohen, B. and Komatsuzaki, A., and Bender, M.B. Electrooculographic
    syndrome in monkeys after pontine reticular formation lesions.
    Arch. Neurol. (Chic.), 18:78-92, 1968.

Cohen, B. and Henn, V. Unit activity in the pontine retcular
    formation associated with eye movements. *Brain Res.*, 46:403-
    410, 1972.

Cohen, B. and Komatsuzaki, A. Eye movements induced by stimulation
    of the pontine reticular formation: evidence for integration
    in oculomotor pathways. *Exp. Neurol.*, 36:101-117, 1972.

Cohen, B., de Jong, V., and Uemura, T, personal communication.

Evinger, C., Fuchs, A.F., and Baker, R. Bilateral lesions of the
    MLF in monkeys: Effect on the horizontal and vertical components
    of voluntary and vestibular induced eye movements. *Exp Brain*
    Res., in press.

Gacek, R.R. Anatomical demonstration of the vestibulo-ocular
    projections in the cat. *Acta-Oto-Laryng.* (Stock.) Suppl.,
    293: 1-63, 1971.

Graybiel, A.M. and Hartwieg, E.A. Some afferent connections of
    the oculomotor complex in the cat: an experimental study
    with tracer techniques. *Brain Res.*, 81:543-551, 1974.

Graybiel, A.M. Direct and indirect pre-oculomotor pathways of the
    brainstem. An autoradiographic study of the pontine reticular
    formation in the cat. Submitted for publication.

Henn, V. and Cohen, B.   Coding of information about rapid eye
    movements in the pontine reticular formation of alert monkeys.
    Brain Res., 108:307-325, 1976.

Highstein, S.M.   The organization of the vestibulo-oculomotor and
    trochlear reflex pathways in the rabbit.   *Exp Brain Res.*, 17:
    285-300, 1973.

Highstein, S.M., Ito, M. and Tsuchiya, T.   Synaptic linkage in the
    vestibulo-ocular reflex pathway of rabbit.   *Exp Brain Res.*,
    13: 306-326, 1971.

Highstein, S.M., Cohen, B. and Matsunami, K.   Monosynaptic projections
    from the pontine reticular formation to the IIIrd nucleus in
    the cat.   *Brain Res.*, 75:340-344, 1974.

Highstein, S.M. and Baker, R.   Excitatory termination of internuclear
    neurons of the abducens nucleus upon medial rectus montoneurons;
    relationship to the syndrome of the MLF.   In preparation.

Keller, E.L.   Participation of medial pontine reticular formation
    in eye movement generation in the monkey.   *J. Neurophysiol.*,
    37:316-332, 1974.

Lorente de No, *Die Labyrinth reflexe auf die Augenmuskeln* Berlin:
    Wiban and Schwarzenberg, 1928.

Maciewicz, R.J., Egan, K., Kaneko, C.R.S. and Highstein, S.M.
    Vestibular and medullary brainstem afferents to the abducens
    nucleus in the cat.   *Brain Res.*, 1977, in press.

Richter, A. and Precht, W.   Inhibition of abducens motoneurons by
    vestibular nerve stimulation.   *Brain Res.*, 11:701-705, 1968.

Schwindt, P.C., Richter, A. and Precht, W.   Short latency utricular
    and canal input to ipsilateral abducens motoneurons, *Brain Res.*,
    60:259-262, 1973.

Tarlov, E.   Organization of vestibulo-oculomotor projections in
    the cat.   *Brain Res.*, 20:159-179, 1970.

Warwick, R.   Oculomotor organization.   In: *The Oculomotor System,*
    (Ed.) M.B. Bender, New York: Harper and Row (Hoeber), pp. 173-
    204, 1964.

THE NUCLEUS PREPOSITUS HYPOGLOSSI

Robert Baker
Department of Physiology and Biophysics
New York University Medical Center
New York, New York

The nucleus prepositus hypoglossi is one of three nuclei found in mammals which have been collectively studied and referred to in the literature as the perihypoglossal nuclei because they surround the hypoglossal nucleus (Brodal, 1952 and 1954; Torvik and Brodal, 1954; Marburg, 1931; and Jermulowicz, 1934). The other two nuclei in the perihypoglossal complex are the nucleus of Roller and the nucleus intercalatus of Staderini. The normal morphological features of the perihypoglossal nuclei have been described in serial transverse sections by Brodal (1952) and Fig. 1 has been reproduced from his original study in the cat.

The caudal part of the perihypoglossal complex contains the nucleus intercalatus of Staderini which is located between the dorsal motor nucleus of the vagus and the hypoglossal nucleus (Fig. 1; 1). At successively rostral levels (2-6) the nucleus intercalatus maintains a position almost centered between the tenth and twelfth cranial nuclei. Near the anterior end of the hypoglossal nucleus (7-8) the nucleus intercalatus expands ventrally to become the nucleus of Roller and continues rostrally as the nucleus prepositus hypoglossi. Each of the three different subdivisions of the perihypoglossal complex has been identified in all species (Barnard, 1949); however, cell size and distribution is not uniform from one animal to another (Barnard, 1949; Brodal, 1952). In addition, the various nuclear subdivisions seemingly fuse imperceptibly with each other in nearly all species investigated (Compare 8-10). In most animals the differentiation between one subdivision of the perihypoglossal nuclei and another has been on the basis of ascertaining a change in cell size at the transition zone and/or in its relationships to other surrounding brain stem

145

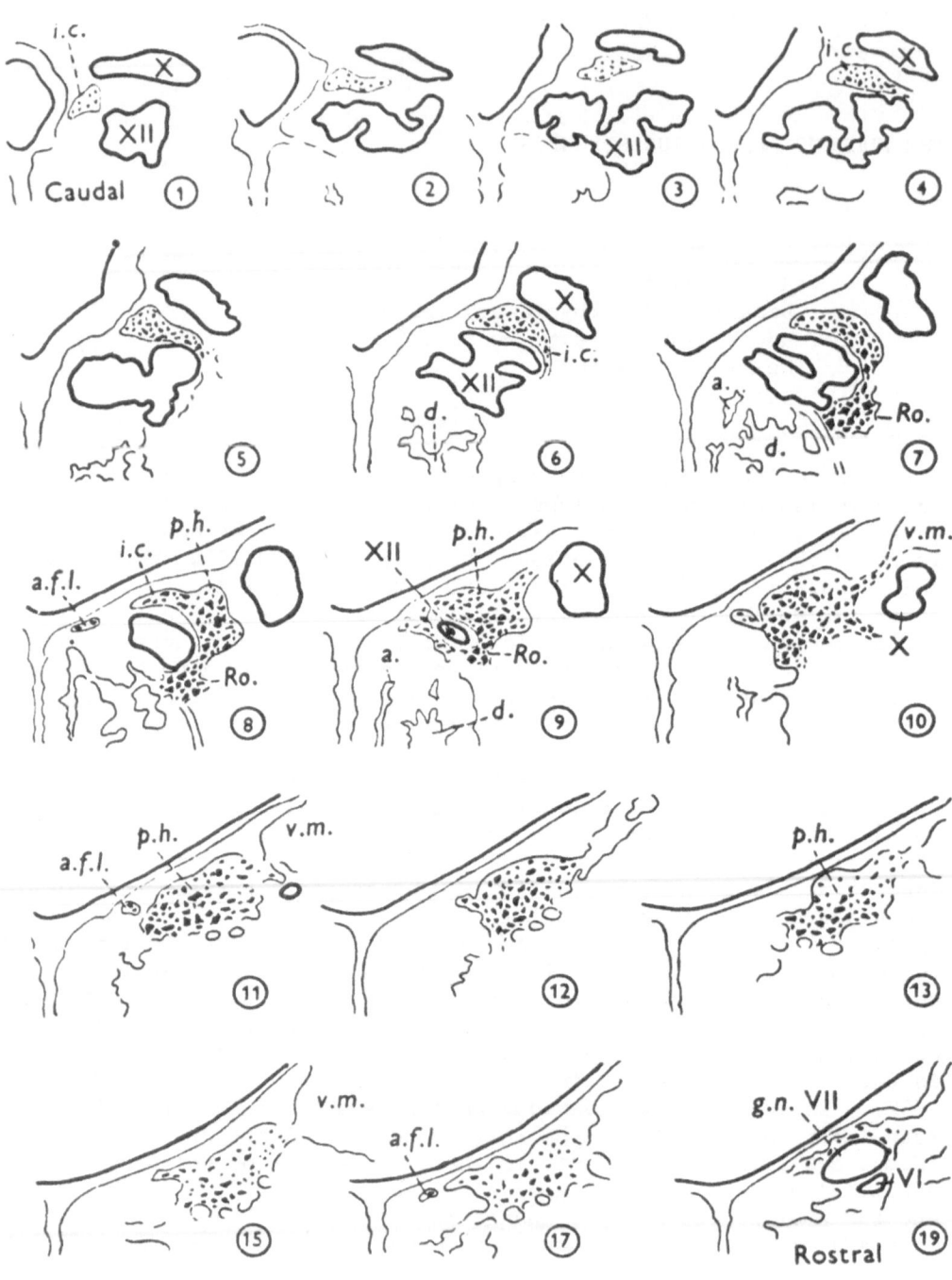

FIGURE 1. Drawings made by means of a projection apparatus of
   transverse Nissl-stained sections through the medulla oblongata
   of a cat 15 days old, showing the topography of the perihypoglossal nuclei. The intervals between the sections represented
   are equal, except for those between 13, 15, 17, and 19
   respectively, which are twice as large. The dots indicate the
   distribution and density of cells of different type. Abbreviations are; *a.*, accessory group of paramedian reticular
   nucleus; *a.f.l.*, annulus fasciculi longtitudinalis posterioris
   of Ziehen; *d.*, dorsal group of paramedian reticular nucleus;
   g.n. VII, genu of facial nerve; *i.c.* nucleus intercalatus of
   Staderini; *p.h.*, nucleus praepositus of Marburg; *Ro.*, nucleus
   of Roller; *v.m.*, medial vestibular nucleus; VI, nucleus of
   abducens nerve; X, dorsal motor nucleus of vagus nerve; XII,
   nucleus of hypoglossal nerve. (Reproduced with the author's
   permission from text-fig. 1 of <u>Brodal, 1952</u>).

nuclei. In the cat, the latter criteria provide a more consistent
landmark than the cellular demarcation (Baker et al., 1975, and
1976).

As one ascends the phylogenetic scale there is an increase in
size, number, and, most noticeably, differentiation of cellular
groups within the perihypoglossal complex (Brodal, 1952; and
Barnard, 1949). This developmental trend not only suggests an
important function for the complex by the time mammalian levels
are attained but also connotes further internal differentiation
within each of the three subdivisions of the perihypoglossal
complex. Since this article emphasizes the prepositus
hypoglossi nucleus in the cat, comparative differences between
species as well as comments on the other two nuclear subdivisions
will not be included (see, however, Brodal, 1952 and 1954, and
Barnard, 1949).

A historical synopsis of how the nucleus prepositus hypoglossi
and its different subdivisions have been recognized and referred
to in prior literature is included below. It should be remembered
that early studies were primarily in man, except Barnard's (1940)
comparative one. The cat is somewhat phylogenetically removed
fom man and some morphological differences are to be expected;
however, according to Brodal (1952) the cat has the same topographical
and cytological features found in man but possibly does not reflect
comparable differentiation within the nucleus itself.

In summary fashion, Marburg's original nucleus praepositus
nervi hypoglossi described in man can be subdivided into a number
of parts. First, there is a caudal area characterized by abundant
large cells found ventrally. This is called the nucleus prepositus
hypoglossi (ph) by Brodal (1952) and is seen in Fig. 1; 8-11. An
apparent rostral density of large cells in close proximity to the
abducens nucleus has suggested another differentiation within the
nucleus. According to Brodal it may be useful to call the anterior
end of the nucleus the supragenualis nervi faciales (Fig. 1; 15-
19). In man, but not in cat, there is a small cell group located
medially which Brodal (1952) has referred to as the nucleus
paramedianus dorsalis (pmd). Finally, in man and probably cat,
there are sparse large cells dorsal to and surrounding the medial
longitudinal fasiculus (Fig. 1; 8, 11, and 17) which have given
rise to the idea of another subdivision of the prepositus nucleus.
Brodal has termed these cells the annulus of the medial longitudinal
fasiculus (afl).

Physiologically it is premature to speculate on any subdivision
of roles within the prepositus because it has not been sufficiently
studied. Up to the present only the posterior magnocellular area
has been extensively investigated physiologically (Baker and

Berthoz, 1975; Baker et al., 1975 and 1976) and these data may be
indicative but possibly not representative because both older and
newer anatomical studies indicate topographical differences in
both afferent and efferent distribution (Brodal, 1952; Walberg,
1961; Ennever-Büttner and Henn, 1976; Angaut and Brodal, 1967;
Alley et al., 1975; Maciewicz et al., 1977; Torvik and Brodal,
1954; Graybiel, 1975; Graybiel and Hartwieg, 1974; Sousa-Pinto,
1970). Thus, we have utilized the expression "prepositus hypoglossi
nucleus", to refer to the whole nucleus but in respect to present
day nomenclature, we prefer the simple term "prepositus nucleus"
first employed by Graybiel and Hartweig (1974).

HISTORICAL NOMENCLATURE OF THE PREPOSITUS NUCLEUS AS REVIEWED
BY BRODAL (1952) (Usage of ph, pmd and afl is in the sense
of Brodal, 1952).

Marburg, 1904
      ph   -   nucleus praepositus nervi hypoglossi
      pmd -   nucleus funiculi teretis (nucleus funiculi or
               eminentiae teretis)

Jacobsohn, 1909
      ph   -   nucleus funiculi
      pmd -   nucleus paramedianus dorsalis

Ziehen, 1934
      ph   -   ventricular part of the nucleus paramedianus
               dorsalis
      pmd -   raphe part of the nucleus paramedianus dorsalis
      afl -   annulus fasciculi longitudinalis posterioris
               of Ziehen

Jermulowicz, 1934
      ph   -   nucleus funiculi teretis
               (rostral) - Kappenker des Facialisknies
               (caudal) - nucleus praepositus
      afl -   annulus fasciculi longitudinalis posterioris
               of Ziehen

Barnard, 1949
      ph   -   nucleus praepositus - in the sense of Marburg
      pmd -   nucleus eminentiae teretis

Brodal, 1952
      ph   -   nucleus praepositus hypoglossi
               (rostral part may be called supragenualis
               nervi faciales)
      pmd -   nucleus paramedianus dorsalis
      afl -   annulus of the medial longitudinal fasciculus

Obviously one of the earliest functions attributed to the prepositus, and to all the perihypoglossal nuclei, was that of the motor control of tongue musculature (Brodal, 1952). On the basis of retrograde chromatolysis, Brodal had evidence that the peri-hypoglossal complex efferents were predominantly precerebellar. Later the work of Torvik and Brodal in 1954 indicated that the cerebellar projection (i.e. the efferent output of the perihypo-glossal complex) was largely to the anterior vermis, pyramis, uvula and fastigial nucleus (Fig. 2). These findings have been confirmed (Alley et al., 1975) but in addition the perihypoglossal nuclei have been shown to project to other areas of the cerebellum, more specifically the flocculus, nodulus and lobules 6 and 7 of the posterior vermis (Fig. 3; Alley et al., 1975; and Alley, unpublished). The failure to observe the vestibulocerebellar projection in earlier studies likely resulted from axon-sparing effects following cerebellar removal due to the now demonstrated dual projection of some prepositus neurons to oculomotor nuclei and cerebellum (Baker and Berthoz, 1975). Following Horseradish Peroxidase (HRP) injections in the vestibulo-cerebellum (Fig. 3; Alley et al., 1975) and oculomotor pathways (Fig. 4; Graybiel and Hartweig, 1974), enzyme reaction products are found in cells distributed throughout the prepositus nucleus. When the latter oculomotor-vestibulo-cerebellar projection is coupled with the demonstration that the vestibulo-cerebellum terminates in the prepositus nucleus (Angaut and Brodal, 1967; and Fig. 5) the diverse data begin to fit together and strongly suggest that the prepositus nucleus might have a function in eye movement. To complete the perspective, Walberg in 1961 had demonstrated that the fastigial nucleus projected onto the prepositus in a fashion similar to its projection onto the medial vestibular nucleus. Specifically, the rostral part of the fastigial nucleus terminated homolaterally in the dorsal prepositus, and the ventral part crossed in the hook bundle and projected to the ventral part of the prepositus nucleus. Finally, vestibular connections from the medial vestibular nucleus were described by Fuse (1914) and Tagaki (1925) but these observations have not yet been studied in detail with recent morphological techniques. It is worth mentioning that much work is required yet to understand the afferent and efferent

---

FIGURE 2.   Summary of the findings of the periphypoglossal nuclei projection to the cerebellum in the cat. The different sub-divisions of the perihypoglossal nuclei are labelled with different symbols and all project on the same cerebellar areas. Note a preponderance of homolateral connections. Additional abbreviations not included in Figure 1: Lob. ant., anterior lobe of vermis; Pyr.,pryamis; Uv., uvula; Nod., nodulus; N.f., nucleus fastigii and C_2, Bolk's lobulus C_2. (Reproduced from text Figure 5 of Torvik and Brodal, 1954).

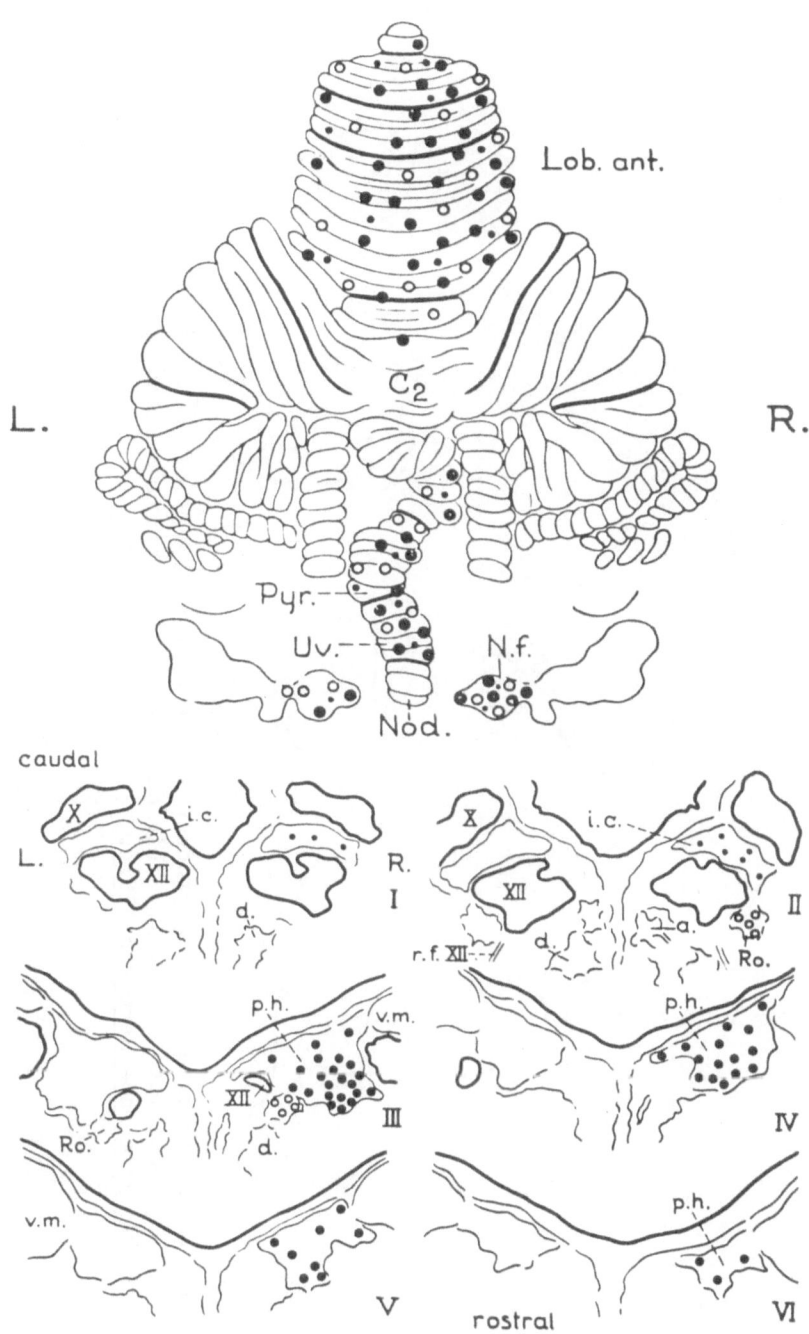

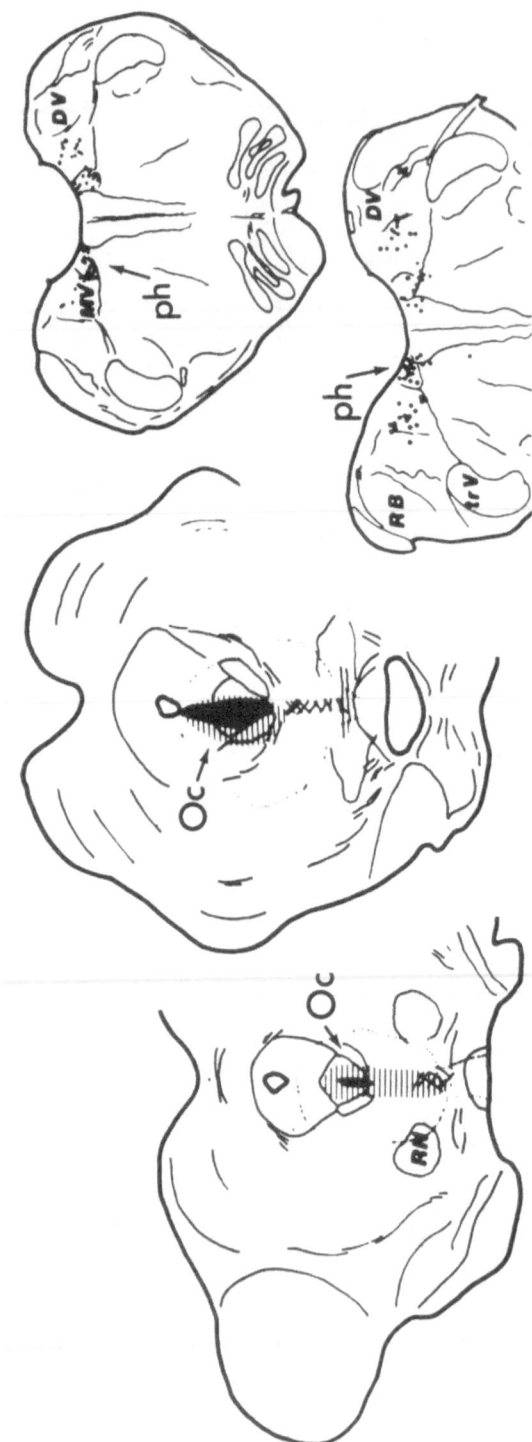

FIGURE 3. Retrograde reaction product in prepositus hypoglossi neurons following HRP injections in the oculomotor complex. This diagram has been provided with permission from the work of <u>Graybiel and Hartweig, 1974.</u>

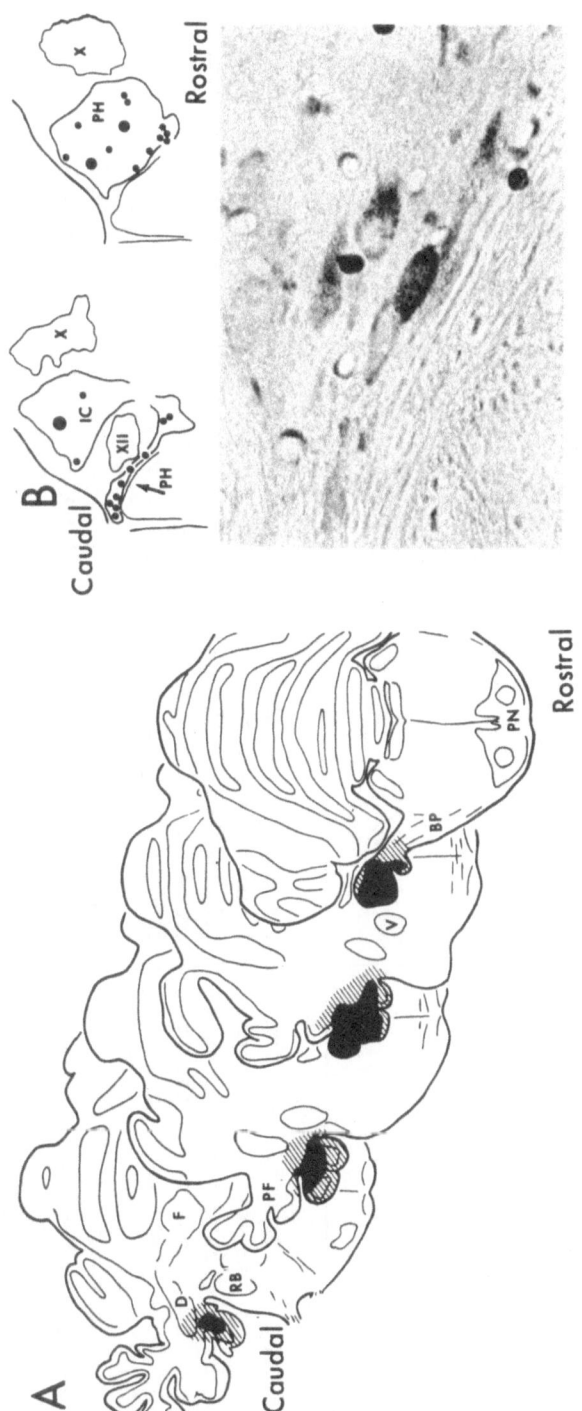

FIGURE 4. Labelling of prepositus hypoglossi neurons following HRP injections into the flocculus. A series of transverse sections on the left in A shows the extent of the HRP injection area and the two insets on the upper right in B indicate schematically the location and number of perihypoglossal neurons filled. In the lower right, a photomicrograph of a cluster of prepositus neurons is shown. This picture was obtained at the level indicated by the arrow in the upper right inset. Abbreviations are similar to those in prior three figures. (Unpublished data reproduced with permission of K. Alley, 1977).

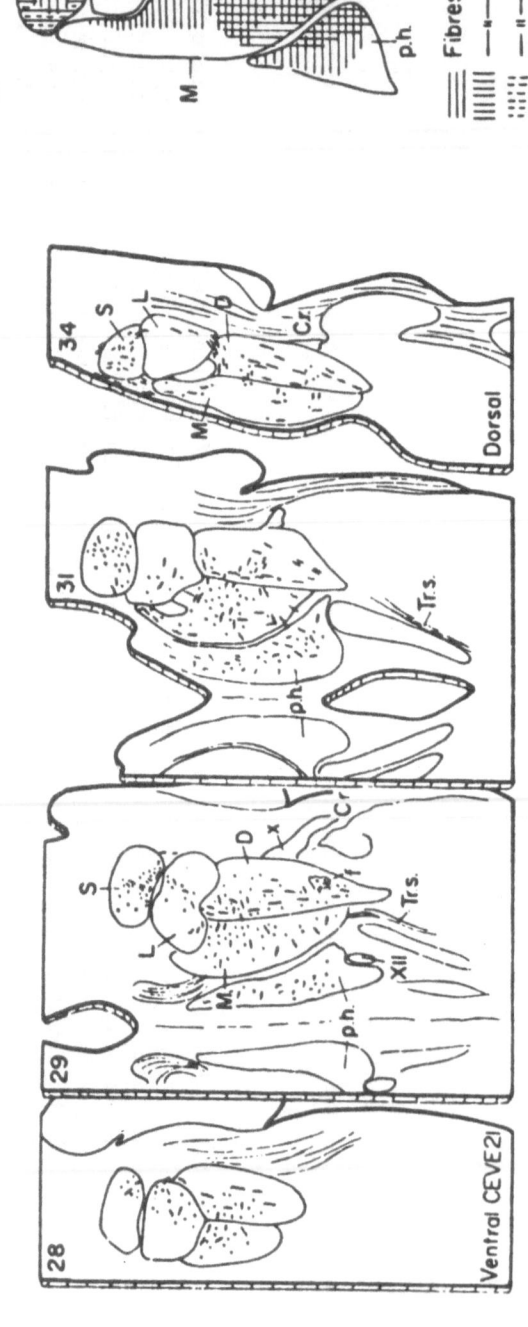

FIGURE 5. Drawings of horizontal sections (A) through the brainstem showing the degeneration in the vestibular nuclei and the prepositus hypoglossi nucleus following a lesion in the homolateral flocculus (not illustrated). The schematic diagram on the right (B) summarizes the findings of the study from which this figure was abstracted. The distributions within the vestibular nuclei of afferents from the flocculus, the nodulus and the uvula are shown by different symbols. Additional abbreviations are: Tr.s, tractus solitarius; C.r, corpus restiforme; f, cell group f in the descending vestibular nucleus; x, small cell group x of Brodal and Pompeiano; S, L, M, and D are the superior, lateral, medial, and descending vestibular nuclei respectively. (Summarized from Fig. 4 and 9 of Angaut and Brodal, 1967).

organization of the prepositus nucleus; even so, the aforementioned HRP studies were successful in initiating a number of new
electro- and neurophysiological investigations. In this paper,
the results from the new prepositus studies are summarized and in
addition, they are discussed in perspective to prior literature
with the overall intent of prompting more work.

In the first series of electrophysiological experiments, we
placed stimulating electrodes on the cerebellar peduncles and
within the oculomotor nuclei in order to antidromically identify
neurons in the prepositus nucleus (Fig. 6A). Generally field
potential depth profiles were complex to interpret due to the
superficial and strategic, in respect to MLF and vestibular nuclei,
location of this nucleus; however, we were able to easily find
antidromically activated cells throughout the anterior-posterior
extent of the prepositus nucleus (Fig. 6B). Some cells were
antidromically activated from the cerebellum and the oculomotor
complex, (Baker and Berthoz, 1975) yet these physiological experiments,
like the HRP ones (Graybiel and Hartwieg, 1974, Fig. 4) did not
reveal the nature of the termination in the cerebellum or the
oculomotor complex. In addition, they could not indicate the
oculomotor or cerebellar source for both the excitation and
inhibition found in all prepositus neurons preceding and following
the antidromic activation of these cells (Baker and Berthoz, 1975
and in preparation).

One of the more surprising findings in our studies of the
prepositus nucleus was the strong vestibular afferent input (Baker
and Berthoz, 1975). The most common intracellular finding in
prepositus neurons was a disynaptic EPSP from the contralateral
vestibular nerve (Fig. 6C) and a disynaptic IPSP from the ipsilateral
vestibular nerve (Fig. 6D). The opposite pattern, i.e. reciprocal
consisting of ipsilateral excitation and contralateral inhibition
was observed, but infrequently. Either bilateral vestibular
inhibition or excitation were also found in a few prepositus
neurons. The aforementioned electrophysiological results from
vestibular stimulation were mostly obtained from the posterior
magnocellular part of the prepositus nucleus and little detail was
obtained concerning topographical organization of the vestibular
input. In another experimental paradigm both inhibitory and
excitatory secondary vestibular neurons projecting to the oculomotor
nuclei were shown to send axon collaterals to the prepositus
nucleus (See Fig. 8; Baker et al., 1977 a and b). Utilizing a
terminology developed by Duensing and Schaefer (1958) and popularized
by Shimazu and Precht (1965), the prior mentioned vestibular
synaptic profiles would be consistent with finding type I-IV
responses following either horizontal or vertical angular acceleration.
In a recent study utilizing horizontal vestibular rotation (Blanks
et al., 1977) it was observed that 60% of prepositus neurons were

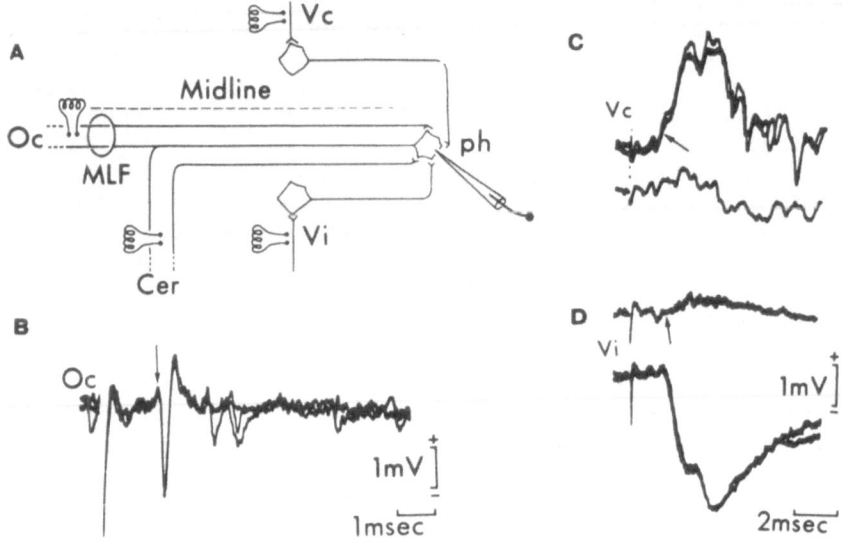

FIGURE 6. Extra- and intracellular records from prepositus hypoglossi neurons following vestibular and oculomotor stimulation.
   A, a schematic diagram showing the sites stimulated and
   synaptic connections established in these experiments. B,
   extracellular record of antidromic activation of the prepositus
   neuron following oculomotor (Oc) stimulation, C, contralateral
   vestibular (Vc) and D, ipsilateral vestibular (Vi) induced
   EPSP and IPSP in a prepositus hypoglossi neuron. The arrows
   point out synaptic latencies of 1.4 msec for the EPSP and
   1.6 msec for the IPSP. (Modified from Baker and Berthoz,
   1975).

type II (i.e., respond like abducens motoneurons on the same side)
and 40% were type I. The preponderance of type II neurons reflect
the contralateral EPSP and ipsilateral IPSP described previously.
In the studies reported by Blanks et al., 1977, horizontal sinusoidal
angular acceleration was utilized to compare the gain and phase of
prepositus neurons with that found in vestibular and abducens
motoneurons (Shimazu and Precht, 1965; and Precht et al., 1967).
In the mid frequency range there was little difference in either
phase or gain for type I and type II cells but the phase lag
regarding head acceleration placed the activity of the prepositus
neurons as somewhat lagging the vestibular but leading the abducens
motoneuron activity.

    In contrast, the response of prepositus neurons to steps of
constant angular acceleration was somewhat different from that of
vestibular neurons. As shown in Fig. 7 (upper record) constant
angular acceleration of $5^{\circ}/sec^2$ lasting for 20 seconds produced a
tonic increase in discharge rate at the onset of the step. The
tonic discharge increased to a steady level, was nonadapting and
the rates of increase in discharge and falloff (i.e. the time
constant) were equal. In this respect the response profiles of
prepositus and vestibular neurons are comparable, but in contrast
vestibular neurons usually showed an exponential increase in rate
of discharge rather than the linear increase found for prepositus
neurons (see Shimazu and Precht, 1965; and Blanks et al., 1977).

    In contrast to the aforementioned response profile, many
prepositus neurons showed an asymmetrical time constant for the
increase of activity as compared to the falloff in response (Fig.
7, lower record). The asymmetry in time constant was proportional
to the magnitude of the stimulus. If the data are viewed collectively,
then phenomena such as linear rate of rise in neuronal activity,
the askewness in the step response, the phase information from the
sinusoidal and other analyses (Blanks et al., 1977) all suggest
that the prepositus nucleus might be a suitable place to envision
the operation of a brain stem integrator. A neuronal operation
resulting in integration has been theorized to be both necessary
and sufficient for the central coding of eye position (Robinson,
1975). In the last series of experiments to be described in this
paper, the activity of prepositus neurons in the alert animal will
in fact be shown to be correlated with changes in eye position
induced by voluntary, vestibular and/or visually guided eye
movement activity. Although displacement in vertical direction
was not tested thoroughly by Blanks et al. (1977), some responses
to changes in angular acceleration were found. This finding
coupled with the one showing neuronal activity related to changes
in vertical eye position (Baker et al., 1975 and 1976, Fig. 10C)
suggest that the prepositus story for both horizontal and vertical
eye movement may be comparable.

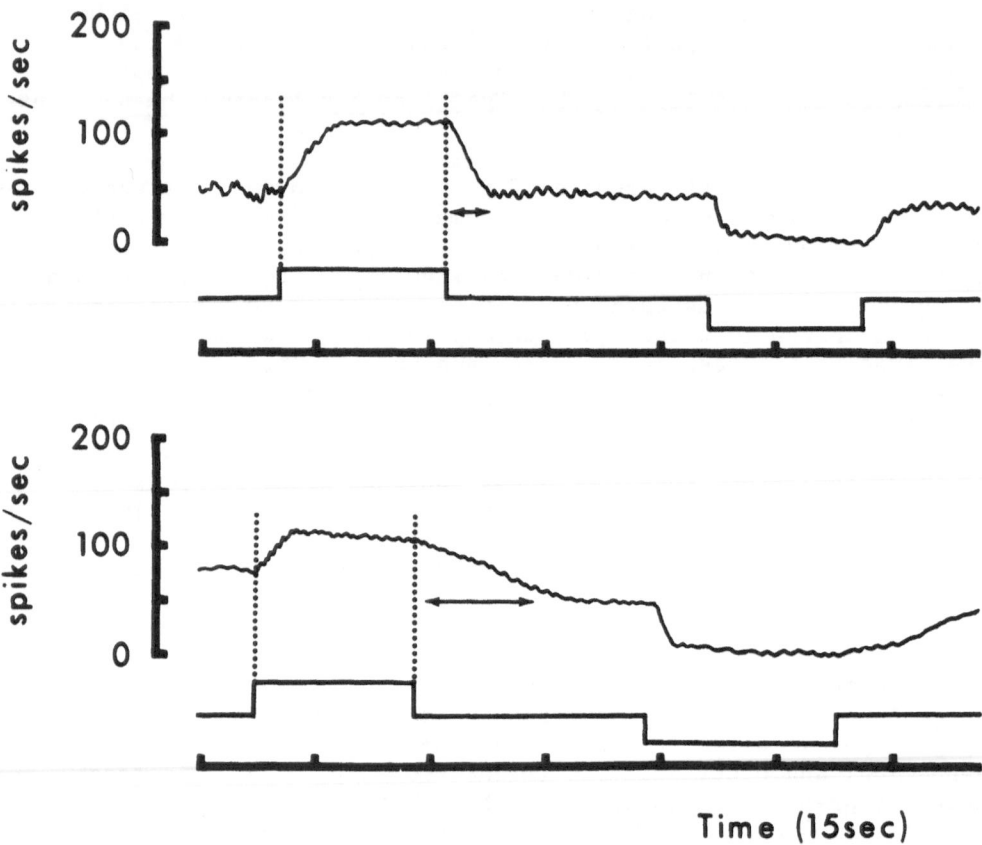

FIGURE 7. The response of two prepositus neurons to constant angular acceleration of $5°/\sec^2$ for 20 seconds. Both cells (upper and lower) were recorded in close proximity to each other within the prepositus hypoglossi nucleus. Explanation in text. (Unpublished data from Blanks et al., 1977).

As another step in analyzing the role for the prepositus hypoglossi nucleus in oculomotor function, experiments were carried out to ascertain whether prepositus neurons terminated directly on (a) oculomotor neurons; (b) in an inhibitory and excitatory fashion, and; (c) in an ipsi or contralateral pathway. In a lengthy series of experiments (Baker et al., 1977 a and b) stimulating electrodes were situated near the anterior end of the ipsi-and contralateral prepositus hypoglossi nucleus and intra- or extracellular records were obtained from all ocular motor subdivisions except for the abducens (Fig. 8). Utilizing the trochlear nucleus as a typical or representative motoneuron for the purpose of this review, the prepositus projection may thus be contrasted simultaneously with the extremely powerful vestibular excitatory and inhibitory input to trochlear motoneurons. As shown in the lower part of Figure 8, stimulation of the fourth cranial nerve in the orbit produces a large antidromic field potential (Tro) when the microelectrode is situated in the center of the trochlear nucleus. Stimulation of the contralateral vestibular nerve (Vc) generated an excitatory (negative) field potential and the ipsilateral vestibular nerve (Vi) a positive inhibitory potential. If the ipsilateral prepositus hypoglossi nucleus (iph) is stimulated only a negative field potential is produced in the trochlear nucleus. This suggested the prepositus projection to be solely excitatory, and accompanying intracellular records obtained from trochlear motoneurons exhibited membrane depolarization with an average latency of about .7-.8 msec indicating monosynaptic excitation (Fig. 9). However, intra-cellular records from motoneurons following chloride injection demonstrated the presence of both short latency excitation and inhibition (Baker et al., 1977 a and b). Since a simple inter-pretation of these results could be compromised by unintentional stimulation of the axon collaterals from inhibitory and excitatory vestibular neurons projecting into the prepositus nucleus (Fig. 8 diagram and Baker et al., 1977a) and/or inadvertent spread of the stimulus current from the stimulation site (near the MLF) to the output of the bilateral vestibular nuclei, we studied cats with chronic lesions separating the bilateral vestibular nucleus from the prepositus as well as animals in which the secondary vestibular projection to the trochlear nucleus was interrupted. Deep bilateral sagittal lesions often compromised the blood supply to the prepositus nucleus and asymmetrical lesions were utilized in order to obtain viable brainstems. In such cases, stimulation of the prepositus hypoglossi nucleus produced only monosynaptic excitatory potentials in trochlear motoneurons but with a longer latency (about 1 msec).

Summarizing the experiments to date, it is worth noting first that only excitatory post synaptic potentials have been found in all ocular motor sub-groups following prepositus stimulation. In addition, this excitation was predominantly elicited from ipsilateral

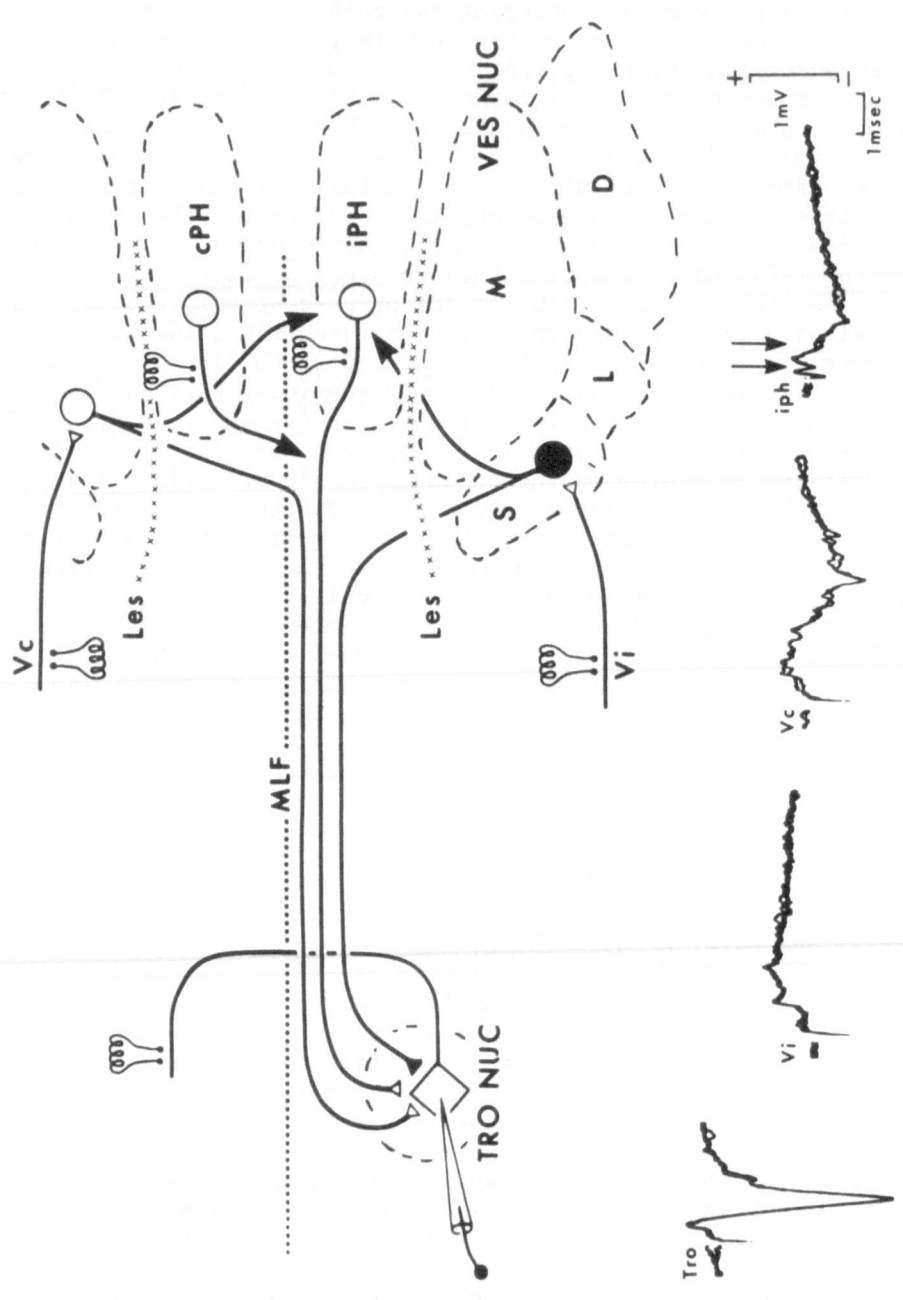

FIGURE 8. A schematic diagram (A) showing the pathways and
    stimulation points for the experimental series studying the
    prepositus hypoglossi projection to trochlear motoneurons.
    Open cells and axon terminals are excitatory, filled ones
    inhibitory, and those with arrows indicate likely projections.
    B: extracellular field potentials recorded near the center of
    the trochlear nucleus. The records from left to right were
    obtained following Tro (5xThr), Vc and Vi (2xThr) and iph
    (3xThr) electrical stimulation. (Summarized from Baker
    et al., 1977a).

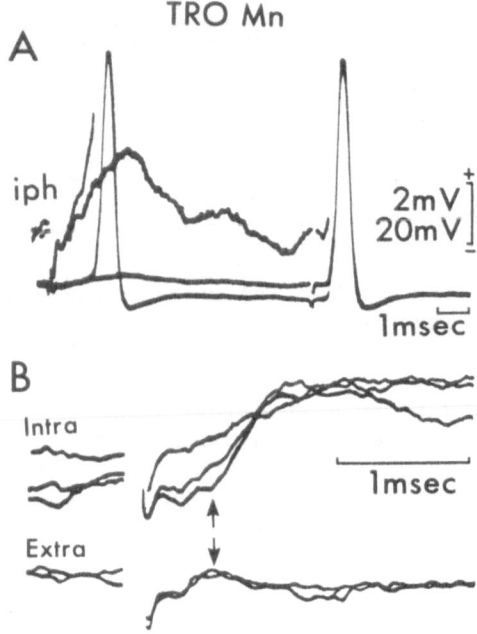

FIGURE 9. Intracellular potentials from a trochlear motoneuron
following stimulation of the prepositus hypoglossi nucleus.
A: EPSP in a Tro Mn following iph (2xThr) and Tro (antidromic response) stimulation. The upper record is AC coupled
high gain and the lower one a DC coupled low gain response.
B: Arrows indicate latency for extra- and intracellularly
recorded depolarization to be 0.7 msec. (Modified from
Baker et al., 1977a).

stimulation sites. Finally, the magnitude of the synaptic potentials were not comparable to the vestibular excitation in any subgroup of ocular motor neurons, thereby suggesting the prepositus hypoglossi termination to be less potent than the vestibular. The latter observation tends to detract from the hypothesis that the prepositus nucleus has a major role in oculomotor function but this finding is counterbalanced by the multiple interactions the prepositus has with brain stem and cerebellar areas already shown to be significant for oculomotor organization.

The most relevant data obtained to date speaking for a role of the prepositus hypoglossi nucleus in eye movement is that observed in the alert animal during voluntary and vestibular induced eye movements (Baker et al., 1975 and 1976). Vestibular induced movements are produced by rotating an animal with its head fixed on a vestibular rate table and optokinetic or pursuit movements can be visually induced by illuminating a large cylindrical projection screen in front of the animal. Microelectrode access to the prepositus hypoglossi nucleus is through the posterior vermis (Fig. 10).

Thus far, we have found two classes of neuronal response in the prepositus hypoglossi nucleus which have been referred to in prior literature as burst-tonic and tonic (Luschei and Fuchs, 1972). The burst-tonic type of activity is shown for a neuron participating in horizontal eye movement (Fig. 10, B) and for a neuron responding to vertical eye movement (Fig. 10, C). The burst response is evident during the saccade and it usually preceded the onset of change in the EOG signal by 6-10 msec. All of the prepositus neurons that respond in a burst-tonic fashion do so similarly for any vestibular or visually guided eye movement. The detailed analysis required to ascertain whether any part of the response pattern is partial to the vestibular or visually evoked movement (see Keller and Daniels, 1975; and Keller, 1974) has not been carried out.

A complete profile of vestibular and optokinetic induced eye movements correlated with the activity of a prepositus neuron during changes in horizontal eye position are shown in Figs. 11 and 12. The monotonic changes in firing frequency of this tonic neuron during voluntary changes in eye position are shown in Fig. 11A. In part B, stimulation of the right vestibular nerve produced successive changes in eye position to the left (see horizontal EOG and arrows) and a pause in the activity of the neuron proportional to the change in eye position. In Fig. 12, the responses of the neuron to OKN with the drum moving from right to left (in A), from left to right (in B) and during one cycle of horizontal vestibular rotation (.15 Hz and 15° amplitude) are shown in C. For comparative physiological reasons, it is pertinent to point out that recordings in the posterior brain stem behind the abducens nucleus in the

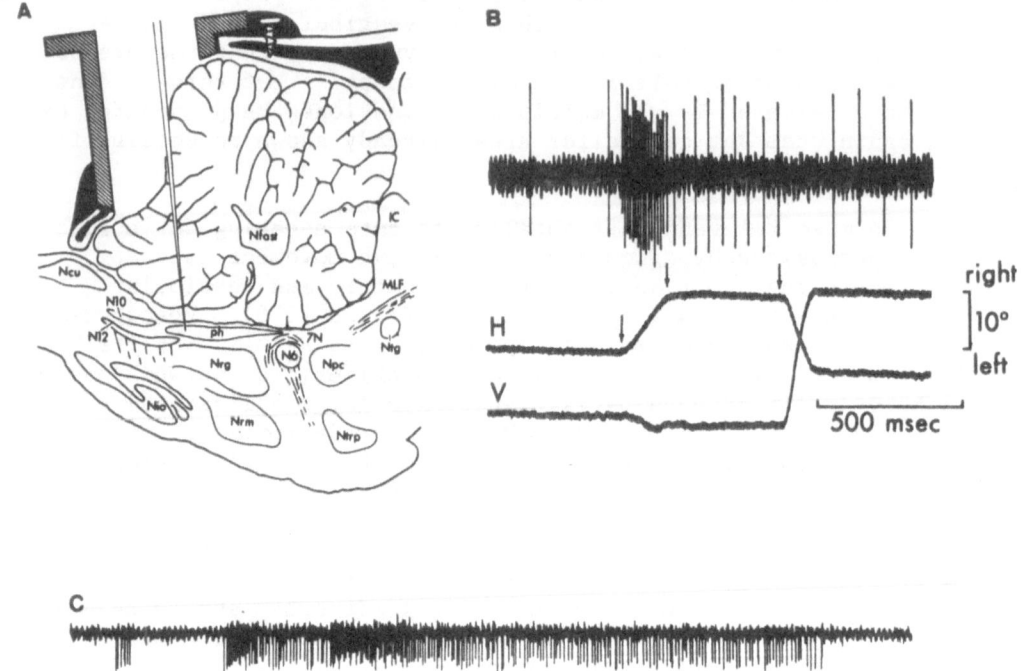

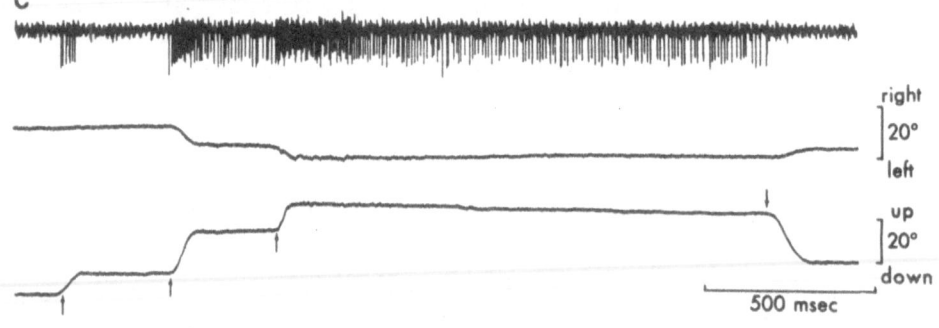

FIGURE 10. Representative activity from two prepositus neurons
during voluntary horizontal and vertical eye movement. The
diagram on the left shows access to the prepositus hypoglossi
nucleus in the alert cat paradigm. New abbreviations are:
Ncu, cuneate nucleus; Nrg, nucleus reticularis gigantocellularis;
Nrtp, nucleus reticularis tegmenti pontis; Ntg, ventral
tegmental nucleus; Nio, inferior olivary nucleus; and IC,
inferior colliculus. B, a prepositus neuron correlated with
horizontal eye movement (on direction *right*) and in C, a cell
correlated with vertical eye movement (on direction *up*).
Arrows indicate the onset and termination of saccade related
activity. (Selection from Baker, et al., 1976.

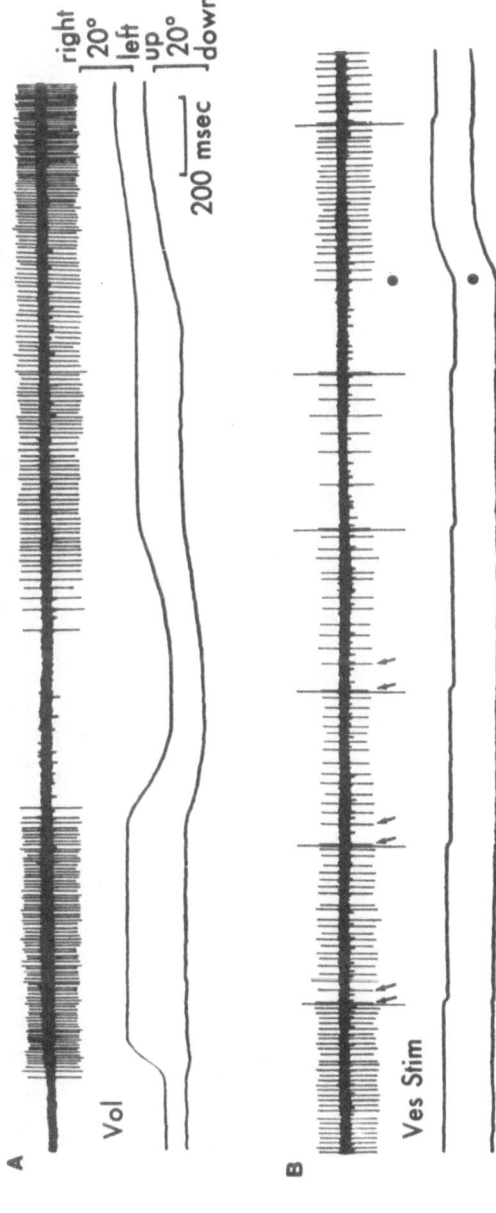

FIGURE 11. The behavior of a prepositus neuron (right brainstem) exhibiting sensitivity to changes in eye position towards the right during a variety of eye movements (See also Figure 12). A, neuronal response during voluntary saccades and pursuit eye movements. B, activity of the unit during isolated double shock stimulation of the right horizontal canal ampulla (2xThr). The stimulation produced stepwise eye displacements (about 2°) toward the left accompanied by a pause in unitary activity (arrows). With successive steps in eye position to the left, the frequency of the unit decreased and a spontaneous saccade (filled dots) to the right reset the position of the eye in the orbit and restored the discharge rate of the prepositus neuron. (Unpublished data, Baker and Gresty).

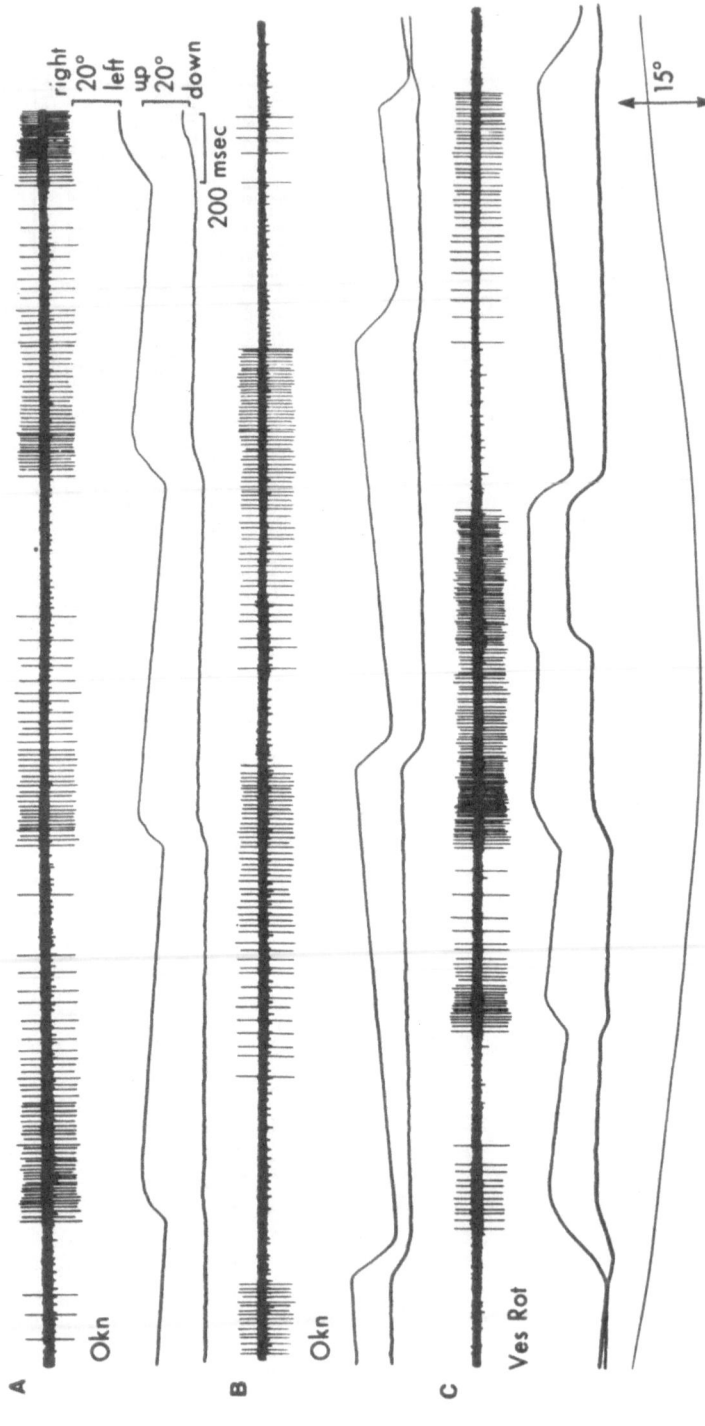

FIGURE 12. Behavior of the prepositus neuron shown in Figure 11 during optokinetic nystagmus induced by stripes moving at 40°/sec in the visual field of the animal towards the left (A) and the right (B). C: Typical behavior of the unit during sinusoidal oscillation of the animal in yaw in darkness. (Unpublished data, Baker and Gresty).

monkey resulted in two classes of responses, namely, horizontal burst-tonic and horizontal tonic neurons (Luschei and Fuchs, 1972). Histologically this is the location of the prepositus hypoglossi nucleus in the primate and it is suggestive that the types of responses observed in the primate were similar to the ones reported herein for the cat. It should be noted, however, that both upward and downward burst-tonic and tonic neurons have been described in the prepositus hypoglossi nucleus in the cat (Baker et al., 1976) but comparable recordings have not yet been obtained in the primate. Although vertical neurons were less numerous than horizontal ones in the study of alert (Baker et al., 1975 and 1976) and lightly anesthetized (Blanks et al., 1977) animals, it is worth noting that the searching stimulus, visual or vestibular, in both experiments was primarily horizontal rather than vertical.

A number of bursting cells (i.e. those in which the discharge rate is not related to eye position) have been observed in either the region of the ventral prepositus hypoglossi nucleus or the dorsal medullary brain stem reticular formation (Gresty and Baker, 1976). These cells burst with horizontal and/or vertical saccades. Some are unidirectional but more commonly they are bidirectional (Fig. 13). The bidirectionality of the burst response is especially noticeable during vestibular induced nystagmus following rotation (Fig. 13B, dots). A more interesting observation with this class of cells was that they nearly all had clear visual receptive fields when examined during long periods of fixation in the cat (Gresty and Baker, 1976). The visual receptive fields were large, eccentrically located, and thus, correspond to the criteria which has been established for receptive fields of superior colliculus neurons (Straschill and Hoffman, 1969). The latter finding is not unreasonable because the superior colliculus terminates densely on the posterior pontis oralis and caudalis areas of the paramedian pontine reticular formation extending as far back as the prepositus hypoglossi nucleus (Kawamura et al., 1974). This observation provides the basis for a visual-vestibular role for the prepositus hypoglossi nucleus. Even so, another group of cells, situated close to the prepositus hypoglossi nucleus and once again slightly ventral are very sensitive to neck displacement (Gresty and Baker, 1976). In this respect, a recent demonstration that precerebellar prepositus neurons receive substantial spinal input could be offered as a basis to suggest an additional role for the prepositus in head and/or neck displacement. In any event, the location of a variety of neuronal responses (such as the burst-tonic, tonic, bursting, displacement, etc.) all situated within close proximity (0.1mm) is challenging for future experimental studies. The diversity of information available within a localized region correlates well with the results of HRP injections in both the oculomotor and cerebellar areas (see Fig. 3 and 4) in that labelled

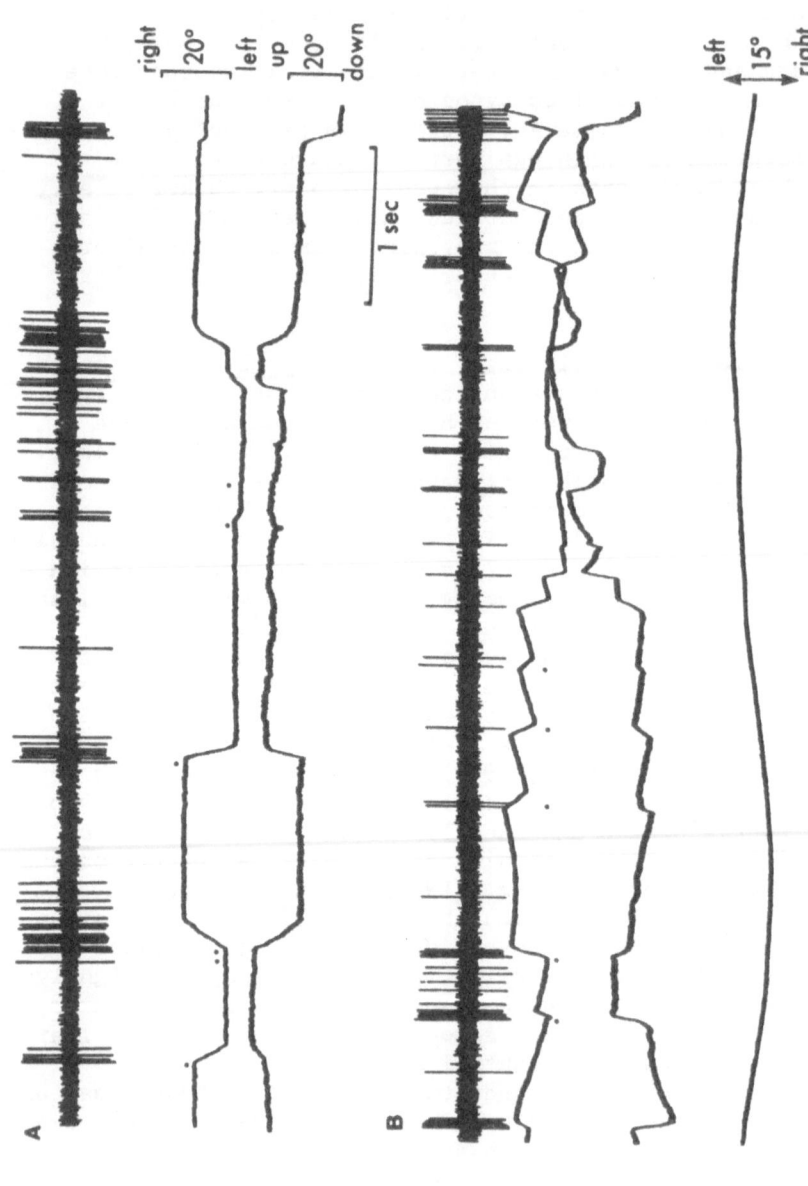

FIGURE 13. The behavior of the prepositus neuron which fires with a burst for both left and rightward eye movements during voluntary saccades (A) and the quick phase of vestibular nystagmus produced sinusoidal oscillation in yaw (B). Dots emphasize bidirectionality of the burst response. This unit was recorded in the ventral part of the right prepositus hypoglossi nucleus. (Unpublished data from Baker and Gresty).

cells are not distributed uniformly throughout the prepositus nucleus but are found in clusters. These findings should be taken into consideration in ascertaining any functional role for the prepositus hypoglossi nucleus.

Although the prepositus hypoglossi nucleus has been sparsely investigated, its relationship to the cerebellar cortex, vestibular and fastigial nuclei, could at first glance more closely tie its activity with a motor and/or regulatory role of the vestibulo-cerebellum. In close similarity with all other immediate prenuclear oculomotor structures thus far investigated, prepositus neurons respond during all types of eye movements (Luschei and Fuchs, 1972; Skavenski and Robinson, 1973; Baker and Gresty, 1976; Keller and Daniels, 1975; Miles, 1974). Our observations that prepositus neurons are directionally selective, except the bursters, and as a population exhibit a strikingly high position threshold (i.e. most active during eccentric gaze) are interesting but not yet that useful. For instance, even though there is gaze nystagmus on attempted eccentric maintained eye positions following MLF lesions (Evinger et al., 1977) it is not possible to attribute such a deficit to a prepositus insufficiency because identified secondary vestibular neurons (Baker and Gresty, 1976; Miles, 1974; Keller and Daniels, 1975) and reticular neurons (Keller, 1974; and Luschei and Fuchs, 1972) also exhibit eye position sensitivity. In conclusion it might be possible to relegate some, but not all, of the eye position function to either the vestibular, reticular or prepositus neuronal population. Data analysis has not progressed to a point where it is possible to determine if the rate-position or rate-velocity curves are different for visual or vestibular induced eye movement. In similar respect, the presence of burst-tonic cells, and thus saccadic information, in a population of prepositus neurons (as well as vestibular and reticular) is also difficult to conceptualize in terms of oculomotor function at the present time.

On the other hand, there is good reason to believe that the prepositus hypoglossi nucleus is likely to be associated with some mid-brain visual mechanism due to its extensive connections with the superior colliculus, pretectal nuclei, accessory ocular nuclei and mesencephalic-pontine reticular formation (Kawamura et al., 1974; Hoddevick et al., 1976; Graybiel, 1975; Ennever-Büttner and Henn, 1976; Hyde, 1964). A visual behavioral role for the hindbrain was suggested long ago in neurological literature following observations of the effect of electrical stimulation of the superior colliculus on induced eye movement (Faulkner and Hyde, 1958). Stimulation of certain collicular regions has been known to produce saccades directed towards a visual receptive field plotted for the very same tectal area (Robinson, 1972a; Apter, 1946; and Straschill and Rieger, 1973). Anatomical studies of efferent projections from the tectum indicate that oculomotor neurons do not receive

direct tectal projections (Altman and Carpenter, 1961; and Kawamura
et al., 1974). If visual motor responses are to reach the posterior
brain stem then they must traverse either the tecto-reticular
(Kawamura and Brodal, 1973) or the tectopontine cerebellar route
(Kawamure et al., 1973). Evidence for a brain stem, tectal to
prepositus, path emerged from the stimulation and lesion experiments
of Hyde and Elliason (1957) and were summarized by Hyde in 1964 in
the form of a diagram shown in Fig. 14. These authors collectively
provide plausible evidence for a descending path from the colliculus
to the ipsilateral mesencephalic reticular formation that decussated
before descending laterally in the pontine brain stem but passed
through the posterior medulla (prepositus hypoglossi nucleus?) to
reach the medial rectus and abducens motoneurons (Fig. 14). In
this series of experiments, Hyde and her colleagues claimed that a
lesion in any part of the aforementioned pathways blocked collicular
evoked eye movement. In the monkey, visual tracking is blocked by
similar lesions in the prepositus hypoglossi nuclei (Uemura and
Cohen, 1973). Furthermore, a reciprocal inhibitory and excitatory
synaptic potential has been recorded in abducens motoneurons
following tectal stimulation (Precht et al., 1974) which (in part)
corroborates the pathways as suggested by Hyde in 1964.

These experimental results, when coupled with the newer ones,
provide a basis for suggesting a visuo-motor pathway related to
some facet of visually induced eye movement through the prepositus
hypoglossi nucleus. Such a hypothesis becomes even more likely by
recent data indicating the role played by the flocculus in visual
tracking (Miles and Fuller, 1976). Experimentally the visuo-motor
hypothesis is worth testing in considerable detail because of the
extensive reciprocal flocculus-prepositus hypoglossi interaction.

FIGURE 14. The collicular-ocular motor pathways as indicated by
    lesion studies in the encéphale isolé. After decussation,
    impulses from the colliculus descend through the lateral
    pontine tegmentum in a compact bundle. Placement of a small
    lesion at A in the diagram blocks left superior colliculus
    evoked eye movement. Caudally, impulses traverse the medial
    reticular substances of the medulla and a lesion at B in the
    right medulla abolishes oculomotor responses to collicular
    stimulation. A lesion at B was without effect on oculomotor
    responses to occipital cortical stimulation. A lesion at C
    in the right MLF abolished adduction to the right. Abbre-
    viations: LMR, left medial rectus muscle; RLR, right lateral
    rectus muscle; III, IV, VI, oculomotor, trochlear and abducens
    nuclei; MED, medial reticular substance of medulla; MLF, medial
    longitudinal fasciculus. (Copy of Figure 5.6 reproduced from
    Hyde, 1964).

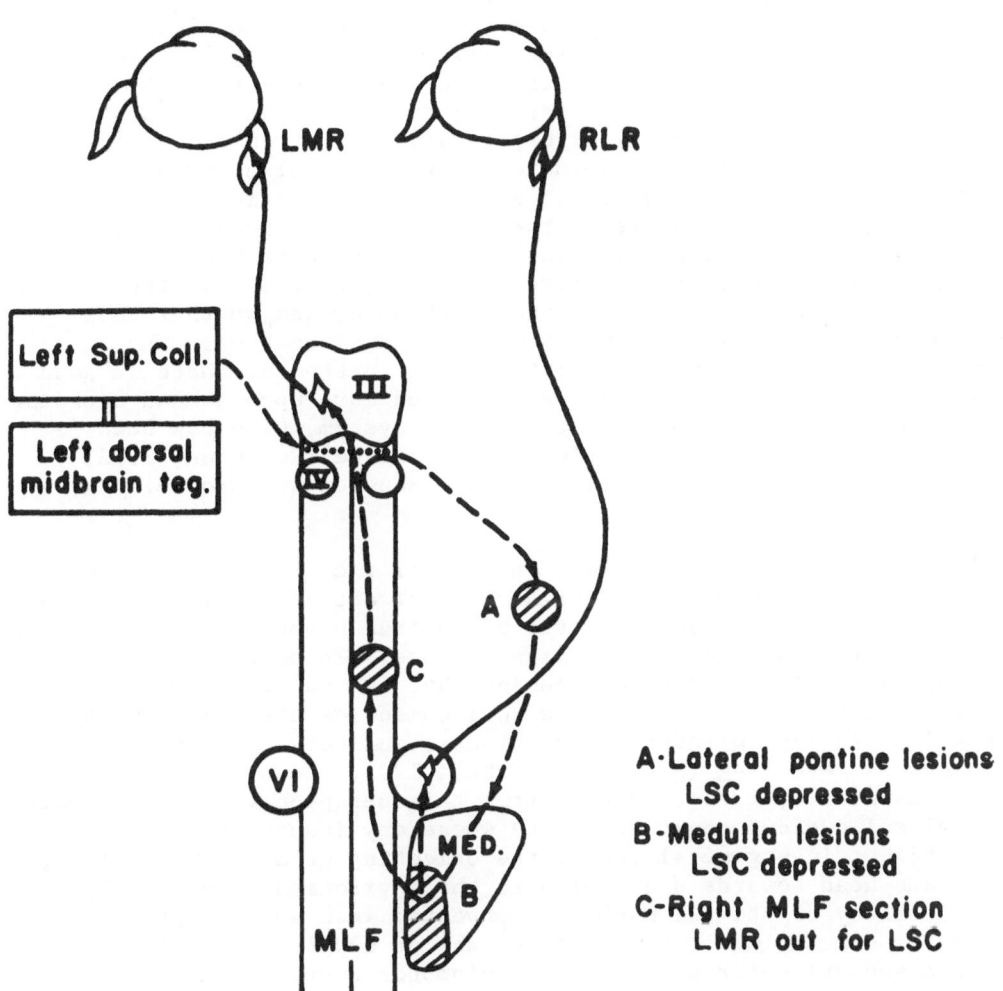

LMR

RLR

Left Sup. Coll.

Left dorsal midbrain teg.

III

IV

VI

MED.

MLF

A

C

B

A·Lateral pontine lesions
　LSC depressed
B·Medulla lesions
　LSC depressed
C·Right MLF section
　LMR out for LSC

In this respect one might speculate whether the aforementioned
vestibulo-cerebello-prepositus-oculomotor relationship is tied to
the problem of retinal-coordinate versus head-coordinate central
eye movement control systems (Robinson, 1975).

In a head coordinate system, initial eye position is held ·to
be important because different movements would occur from various
eye positions. In a retinal coordinate situation, knowledge of
initial eye position is not essential, only the change in eye
position is necessary. These arguments would imply that the
retinotopic signal which is determined by the retina (eye position
minus target position equal error) is available from the superior
colliculus and is already adequate for the retinal coordinate
system. To obtain a head coordinate system the retinotopic signal
must be converted somewhere in the CNS to an appropriate premotor
signal which has encoded eye position in respect to head position.
Given the afferent-efferent organization and location of the
prepositus hypoglossi nucleus, the question arises whether this
area might be the site of such a signal transformation. The
hypothesis has considerable merit because in the cat there is good
evidence that eye movement is indeed based more upon a head coordinate
rather than a retinal coordinate control system which has been
suggested to be more applicable to the primate (Robinson, 1972, a
and b; Straschill and Rieger, 1973; and Roucoux and Crommelinck,
1976).

Recent studies implicating the superior colliculus in visual
guidance of eye movement and/or a shift of attention with facilitation
of eye movement suggests that the prepositus hypoglossi nucleus
could be of even more general significance. In the latter respect,
demonstration in a number of species that the superior colliculus
contains a representation of the environment of the animal with
superimposed maps of surrounding visual, auditory and somatosensory
sources is revealing (Drager and Hubel, 1975; Stein et al., 1975;
Abrahams et al., 1975). Viewed from this perspective, the prepositus
hypoglossi nucleus could be a site where any induced shift of
attention (in a general sense, the orienting of an animal's eyes,
ears and head towards a stimulus in the environment) induced by a
wide variety of stimuli might be converted into an appropriate
premotor command which either initiates or supplements more
direct sensori-motor pathways to oculomotor neurons.

In conclusion, the relatively weak (but direct) prepositus
termination on oculomotor neurons produces little enthusiasm
regarding the hypothesis that the prepositus nucleus may be singularly
sufficient for producing any conjugate eye movement, let alone a
visually-guided one. In spite of this limitation the ubiquitous
influence this posterior brain stem area exercises at many neural
levels might permit it to meet the necessary requirements to do

so. If all the interfaces with other central nuclei (i.e. the
flocculus, vestibular, reticular and ocular nuclei) are considered
to be sufficient in the cat, an animal with poor eye movement,
then given the size of the nucleus in the primate, it seems reasonable
to pursue the idea that the prime role of the prepositus hypoglossi
nucleus is one of a visual-motor nature.

ACKNOWLEDGEMENTS

Supported by USPHS grants EY-02007, NS-13742 and CNRS in Paris.
Permission from my colleagues to include both published and
unpublished material is sincerely appreciated.

REFERENCES

Abrahams, V. C. and Rose, P.K. Projections of extraocular, neck
    muscle, and retinal afferents to superior colliculus in the
    cat: their connections to cells of origin of tectospinal
    tract. *J. Neurophysiol.*, 38:10–18, 1975.

Akert, K. Experimenteller Beitrag betreffs die zentrale Netzhautre-
    presentation in Tectum opticum. *Schweiz. Arch. Neurol.
    Neurochir. Psychiat.*, 64:1–16, 1949.

Alley, K., Baker, R., and Simpson, J.I. Afferents to the vestibulo-
    cerebellum and the origin of the visual climbing fibers in
    the rabbit. *Brain Res.*, 98:582–589, 1975.

Altman, J., and Carpenter, M.B. Fiber projections of the superior
    colliculus in the cat. *J. Comp. Neurol.*, 116:157–178, 1961.

Angaut, P., and Brodal, A. The projection of the 'vestibulocere-
    bellum' onto the vestibular nuclei in the cat. *Arch. Ital.
    Biol.*, 105:441–479, 1967.

Apter, J. T. Projection of the retina on superior colliculus of
    cats. *J. Neurophysiol.*, 8:123–134, 1945.

Baker, R., and Berthoz, A. Is the prepositus hypoglossi nucleus
    the source of another vestibular ocular pathway? *Brain
    Res.*, 86:121–127, 1975.

Baker, R., and Berthoz, A. Vestibular input to the prepositus
    hypoglossi nucleus. *Fed. Proc.*, 34:439, 1975.

Baker, R., Berthoz, A., and Delgado–Garcia, J. Monosynaptic
    excitation of trochlear motoneurons following electrical
    stimulation of the prepositus hypoglossi nucleus. *Brain
    Res.*, 121:157–161, 1977.

Baker, R., and Delgado–Garcia, J. Projection of the prepositus
    hypoglossi nucleus on to the oculomotor nuclei. In pre-
    paration, 1977.

Baker, R., and Gresty, M. Intracellular records from trochlear
    motoneurons and axons of identified secondary vestibular
    neurons in the alert cat during eye movement. *The
    Physiologist*, 19:114, 1976.

Baker, R., Gresty, M., and Berthoz, A. Physiological studies
    establishing a vestibulo-cerebello-oculomotor role for the
    prepositus hypoglossi nucleus. In *Eye Movements and Motion
    Perception* - Ninth Symposium of the Center for Visual Science
    Rochester, N.Y., pp. 39-40, 1975.

Baker, R. Gresty, M., and Berthoz, A. Neuronal activity in the
    prepositus hypoglossi nucleus correlated with vertical and
    horizontal eye movement in the cat. *Brain Res.*, 101:366-
    371, 1976.

Baker, R., and Highstein, S. Physiological identification of inter-
    neurons and motoneurons in the abducens nucleus. *Brain Res.*,
    91:292-298, 1975.

Blanks, R.H.I., Volkind, R. Precht, W., and Baker, R. Responses
    of cat prepositus hypoglossi motoneurons to horizontal angular
    acceleration. In press, *Neuroscience*, 1977.

Brodal, A. Experimental demonstration of cerebellar connections
    from the peri-hypoglossal nuclei (nucleus intercalatus,
    nucleus praepositus hypoglossi and nucleus of Roller) in
    the cat. *J. Anat.* (Lond.), 86:110-120, 1952.

Brodal, A. Cerebellar afferents from the peri-hypoglossal nuclei.
    In: *Aspects of Cerebellar Anatomy*. Ed. by J. Jansen and A.
    Brodal, Oslo: Gunderson, pp. 158-161, 1954.

Büttner-Ennever, J., and Henn, V. An autoradiographic study of the
    pathways from the pontine reticular formation involved in eye
    movements. *Brain Res.*, 108:155-164, 1976.

Dräger, V.C., and Hubel, D.A. Responses to visual stimulation and
    relationship between visual, auditory and somatosensory inputs
    in mouse superior colliculus. *J. Neurophysiol.*, 38:690-713,
    1975.

Duensing, F., and Schaefer, K.P. Die Aktivat einzelner Neuronen
    im Bereich der Vestibulärischkerne bei Horizontalbeschleunig-
    ungen unter besonderer Beruchsichtigung des vestibulären
    Nystagmus. *Arch. Psychiat. Nervenkr.*, 198:225-252, 1958.

Eccles, J.C., Nicoll, R.A., Schwarz, D.W.F., Taborikova H., and
    Willey, T.J. Medial reticular and perihypoglossal neurons
    projecting to the cerebellum. *J. Neurophysiol.*, 39:102-
    108, 1976.

Evinger, C.L., Fuchs, A.F., and Baker, R. Bilateral lesions of the
    medial longitudinal fasciculus in monkeys: Effects on the
    horizontal and vertical components of voluntary and vestibular
    induced eye movements. In press, *Exp. Brain Res.*, 1977.

Faulkner, R.R., and Hyde, J.E. Coordinated eye and body movements
    evoked by brainstem stimulation in decerebrated cats. *J.
    Neurophysiol.*, 21:171–182, 1958.

Fuse, G. Beitrag zur anatomie des Bondens des IV Ventrikels.
    Arb. Hirnanat. Inst. Zurich, 8:213–231, 1914.

Graybiel, A.M. Anatomical pathways in the brainstem oculomotor
    system. In *Eye Movements and Motion Perception* – Ninth
    Symposium of the Center for Visual Science, Rochester,
    N.Y., pp. 37–48, 1975.

Graybiel, A.M., and Hartweig, E.A. Some afferent connections of
    the oculomotor complex in the cat: an experimental study
    with tracer techniques. *Brain Res.*, 81:543–551, 1974.

Gresty, M., and Baker, R. Neurons with visual receptive field, eye
    movement and neck displacement sensitivity within and around
    the nucleus prepositus hypoglossi in the alert cat. *Exp.
    Brain Res.*, 24:429–433, 1976.

Hyde, J.E. Interrelationship from brainstem and cortical areas
    for conjugate ocular movements in cats. In: *The Oculomotor
    System.* ed. Bender, M.B., Harper and Row: N.Y., pp. 141–
    149, 1964.

Hyde, J.E., and Eliasson, S.G. Brainstem induced eye movements in
    the cat. *J. Comp. Neurol.*, 108:139–172, 1957.

Jermulowicz, W. Untersuchungen uber die Kerne am Boden der
    Rautengrube (Nucleus paramedianus, Nucleus eminentae teretis,
    Nucleus praepositus hypoglossi , Kappenkern des Facialisknies)
    Z. Anat. Enwickl.-Gesch., 103:290–302, 1934.

Kawamura, K., and Brodal, A. The tectopontine projection in the
    cat: an experimental anatomical study with comments on
    pathways for teleceptive impulses to the cerebellum. *J. Comp.
    Neurol.*, 149:371–390, 1973.

Kawamura, K., Brodal, A., and Hoddevik, G. The projection of the
    superior colliculus onto the reticular formation of the brain-
    stem. An experimental anatomical study in the cat. *Exp.
    Brain Res.*, 19:1–19, 1974.

Keller, E.L. Participation of medial pontine reticular formation
    in eye movement generation in monkey. *J. Neurophysiol.*,
    37:316-322, 1974.

Keller, E.L., and Daniels, P.D. Oculomotor related interaction
    of vestibular and visual stimulation in vestibular nucleus
    cells in alert monkey. *Exp. Neurol.*, 46:187-198, 1975.

Ladpli, R., and Brodal, A. Experimental studies of commissural and
    reticular formation projections from the vestibular nucleus
    in the cat. *Brain Res.*, 8:65-96, 1968.

Luchei, E.S., and Fuchs, A.F. Activity of brainstem neurons during
    eye movements of alert monkeys. *J. Neurophysiol.*, 35:
    445-461, 1972.

Machiewicz, R.J., Eagen, K., Kaneko, C.R.S., and Highstein, S.M.
    Vestibular and medullary brainstem afferents to the abducens
    nucleus in the cat. In press, *Brain Res.*, 1977.

Marburg, O. Das Dorsale Langsbundel von Schutz – Fasciculus
    periependymalis–und seine Beziehungen zu den Kernen des
    zentralen Hohlengraus. *Arb. Neurol. Inst. Univ. Wien.*,
    33:135-164, 1931.

Miles, F.A. Single unit firing patterns in the vestibular nuclei
    related to voluntary eye movements and passive body rotation
    in conscious monkeys. *Brain Res.*, 71:215-224, 1974.

Miles, F., and Fuller, J.H. Visual tracking and the primate
    flocculus. *Science,* 189:1000-1002, 1975.

Precht, W., Richter, A., and Grippo, J. Responses of neurons in
    cats abducens nuclei to horizontal angular acceleration.
    Pflug. Arch., 309:285-309, 1967.

Precht, W., Schwindt, P.C., and Magherini, P.C. Tectal influences
    on cat ocular motoneurons. *Brain Res.*, 82:27-50, 1974.

Robinson, D.A. Eye movements evoked by collicular stimulation in
    the alert monkey. *Vision Res.*, 12:1795-1808, 1972a.

Robinson, D.A. On the nature of visual–oculomotor connections.
    Invest. Ophthal., 11:497-503, 1972b.

Robinson, D.A. Oculomotor control signals. In *Basic Mechanisms
    of Ocular Motility and Their Clinical Implications.* ed.
    Lennerstrand G. and Bach-y-Rita, P.; Pergamon Press: London
    pp. 337-374, 1975.

Roucoux, A., and Crommelinck, M.   Eye movements evoked by superior
    colliculus stimulation in the alert cat. *Brain Res.*, 106:
    349-370, 1976.

Shimazu, H., and Precht, W.   Tonic and kinetic responses of cat's
    vestibular neurons to horizontal angular acceleration.
    J. Neurophysiol., 28:991-1013, 1965.

Skavenski, A.A., and Robinson, D.A.   Role of abducens neurons in
    vestibulo-ocular reflex. *J. Neurophysiol.*, 36:724-738, 1973.

Sousa-Pinto, A.   The cortical projection onto the paramedian
    reticular and perihypoglossal nuclei (nucleus praepositus
    hypoglossi, nucleus intercalatus and nucleus of Roller)
    of the medulla oblongata of the cat.   An experimental-
    anatomical study. *Brain Res.*, 18:77-91, 1970.

Stein, B.E., Magalhaes-Castro, B., and Kruger, L. Superior colliculus
    visuotopic-somatotopic overlap. *Science,* 189:224-226, 1975.

Straschill, M., and Hoffmann, K.P.   Functional aspects of locali-
    zation in the cats tectum opticum. *Brain Res.*, 13:274-283, 1969.

Straschill, M., and Rieger, P.   Eye movements evoked by focal
    stimulation of the cats superior colliculus. *Brain Res.*,
    59:221-227, 1973.

Tagaki, J.   Studien zur vergleichenden Anatomie des Nucleus vesti-
    buläris triangularis.   I.   Der Nucleus intercalatus und der
    Nucleus praepositus hypoglossi. *Arb. Neurol. Inst. Univ.
    Wein.*, 27:157-188, 1925.

Torvik, A., and Brodal, A.   The cerebellar projection of the peri-
    hypoglossal nuclei (nucleus intercalatus, nucleus praepositus
    hypoglossi and nucleus of Roller) in the cat. *J. Neuropath.
    Exp. Neurol.*, 13:515-527, 1954.

Uemura, T., and Cohen, B.   Effects of vestibular nuclei lesions on
    vestibulo-ocular reflexes and posture in monkeys. *Acta. Oto-
    Laryng. Suppl.*, 315:1-71, 1973.

Walberg, F.   Fastigiofugal fibers to the perihypoglossal nuclei in
    the cat. *Exp. Neurol,* 3:525-541, 1961.

Ziehen, Th.   Centralnervensystem. In: *Bardelebens Handb. Anat.
    Menschen,* 4, pt. 2., Jena: G. Fischer, 1934.

THE NEURAL CONTROL OF SACCADIC EYE MOVEMENTS: THE ROLE OF THE SUPERIOR COLLICULUS

David L. Sparks and Jay G. Pollack
Department of Psychology, The Neurosciences Program
and the School of Optometry
University of Alabama in Birmingham
Birmingham, Alabama

INTRODUCTION

Traditionally, the superior colliculus (SC) has been considered a center for producing reflexive movements of the eyes and head in response to visual stimuli. But the suggestion that the SC is a critical or necessary structure for voluntary or involuntary eye movements has been vigorously disputed (Pasik et al., 1966). In recent years, evidence has accumulated which supports earlier suggestions that the SC is involved in coding the location of an object relative to the fovea and in eliciting saccadic movements which produce foveal acquisition of the object. An alternative hypothesis, that the SC is concerned with shifting attention to specific areas of the visual field, has received experimental support as well.

Major aims in the preparation of this paper were (1) to present a selected review of experiments related to the role of the SC in the control of eye movements, (2) to identify areas in which additional research is needed, and (3) to present speculations concerning specific roles the SC may play in the initiation and execution of saccades. With certain exceptions, data obtained from the monkey (Macaca mulatta) SC has been emphasized. Many important studies have not been referenced, particularly those using cats as subjects. The growing literature related to the effects of early modification of visual experience upon the properties of SC neurons is not reviewed.

Sprague et al., (1973) have recently reviewed the role of the SC and pretectum in visually guided behavior. Also, a report

179

of a Neurosciences Research Program work session of the sensorimotor
function of the midbrain tectum appeared recently (Ingle and
Sprague, 1975).

ANATOMY OF THE SUPERIOR COLLICULUS

This section reviews the anatomy of the SC of the Rhesus
monkey. Non-primate studies are discussed only for comparison or
where they contribute information which is lacking for the monkey.

General Organization

The SC is composed of seven alternating fibrous and cellular
layers. From the surface towards the central gray, these are the
stratum zonale (SZ), stratum griseum superficiale (SGS), stratum
opticum (SO), stratum griseum intermedium (SGI), stratum album
intermedium (SAI), stratum griseum profundum (SGP), and stratum
album profundum (SAP). These strata have recently been divided
into two divisions -- the superficial (SZ, SGS, SO) and deep (SGI,
SAI, SGP, SAP) -- based on differences in their afferents (Lund,
1964; Victorov, 1966) as well as their efferent projections and
functional criteria (Casagrande, et al., 1972, 1974; Harting, et
al., 1973; Schneider, 1969) in several species. These subdivisions
have been extended to the monkey on anatomical grounds (Benevento
and Fallon, 1975) though the functional effects of discrete lesions
confined to either division have not been examined. In general,
the superficial division receives primarily visual afferents and
has efferents destined for several thalamic nuclei. The deep
division receives a multimodal afferent projection and has descending
efferents as well as ascending efferents to several thalamic
nuclei which may or may not also receive fibers from the superficial
division. These relationships are discussed in detail below.

Projections to the Superior Colliculus

Afferents to the superficial division. Axons arising in the
retina and in the visual cortex terminate, for the most part, in
the uppermost layers of the SC (SGS and SZ). These fibers are
arranged on the collicular surface in an orderly manner, with both
the retinal and visual cortical fibers that are responsive to a
given region of the field terminating in corresponding regions of
the colliculus (see Lund, 1972 for references). The representation
of the visual field is not uniform, the central 10 deg occupying
over 30% of the anterolateral collicular surface while the peripheral
visual field is compressed into the remaining area (Cynader and
Berman, 1972).

The contribution of the retina and of the visual cortex to
visually responsive cells in the superficial division has been

given a great deal of consideration in the anatomical literature.
One particular generalization which emerges from these studies is
that in those mammals exhibiting relatively uniform visual acuity
(e.g., the rat or marmot), the retina provides the densest input
to the superficial division while the cortex provides only a minor
contribution. For example, in the rat, Lund (1972) estimates that
the cortex uses less than 1% of the total synaptic space in the
SGS while retinal afferents comprise over 50%. Animals with
uniform retinas have little need for precise saccadic movements
since one region of the retina provides no better visual acuity
than any other region (Wall, 1967). Mammals with retinal special-
izations (e.g., area centralis, fovea) display more voluntary eye
movements and the cortex takes up a larger percentage of synaptic
space compared to the retina, particularly in the representation
of the specialization on the collicular surface. This is seen in
its most extreme form in the primate.

     Hubel et al. (1975) have recently described the distribution
of afferent fibers from the retina to the SC in monkey. In the
most caudal region of the SC (monocular segment) the contralateral
eye projects throughout the SGS. In the area representing the
binocular peripheral visual field, the contralateral input is a
continuous sheet in the upper part of the SGS, while the ipsilateral
input is more ventral. The ipsilateral input appears as small
discontinuous puffs of terminals in transverse sections, which
have recently been shown by Graybiel (1976) to form longitudinal
bands of input when reconstructed from serial sections. More
anteriorly, both the contralateral and ipsilateral inputs thin,
become more dorsally placed and appear, presumably, as alternating
puffs from the two eyes. In the anterolateral region, which
represents the perifoveal and foveal visual field, there is a
"weak, but definite" projection (Hubel et al., 1975). We examined
the distribution of retinal fibers to the SC after intraocular (H^3)
proline injection in one Rhesus monkey (unpublished). Our results
were similar to those reported above, except that we were unable
to detect terminals in the region of the colliculus corresponding
to the central 1 - 2 deg of visual field as described by
Cynader and Berman (1972). A sparse distribution of terminals was
clearly evident in the area corresponding to perifovea. A sparse
projection from retina to the anterolateral region has also been
described by Hendrickson et al., (1970), though degeneration
studies (Lund, 1972; Wilson and Toyne, 1970) and an HRP study
(Bunt et al., 1975) failed to find any evidence for a foveal
retinal input. It is, however, clear that the projection from
retina is greatest from peripheral visual field and drastically
diminished towards the central visual field in monkey.

     Bunt et al., (1975) examined the distribution of ganglion
cells sending afferents to the SGS using the retrograde marker

HRP. They found that no particular group of cells, based upon
cell size, could be discerned and that labeled cells were located,
sparsely, throughout the retina (except in the fovea). By comparison,
cells of all sizes send afferents to the colliculus in the cat,
but there is a marked predominance of small cells (Magalhaes-
Castro et al., 1976). Bunt et al., (1975) also suggest that since
all retinal ganglion cells appeared to send afferents to the
dorsal LGN, those axons terminating in the colliculus were collaterals
of some of these afferents.

In the monkey SC, a major source of visually organized
afferents to the superficial division, particularly in the representation of the central visual field, is from striate cortex (Black
and Myers, 1962; Campos-ortega and Hayhow, 1972; Kuypers and
Lawrence, 1967; Lund et al., 1975; Lund et al., 1972; Myers 1962;
Wilson and Toyne, 1970). The cells of orgin of the corticotectal
projection to SGS appear to be from both large and small pyramidal
type cells in Lund and Booth's (1975) lamina 5 of area 17 (Lund et
al., 1975). The central visual field, represented at the junction
of the lunate and occipital sulci, projects to the anterior
colliculus. That from the horizontal meridian representation
(dorsal convexity of area 17 and bottom of calcarine sulcus)projects
anteriolaterally to posteriomedially on the collicular surface,
and that from the vertical meridian projects medial to lateral on
the colliculus (Wilson and Toyne, 1970). Possible projections
from visual areas 18 and 19 to SGS do not appear to have been
studied in monkey with contemporary neuroanatomical methods,
though such projections to cat SGS are known (Garey et al., 1968;
Palmer et al., 1972; Gilbert and Kelly, 1975). It is possible
that area 18 projects to the SGS only indirectly in monkey.

Though the major sources of input in the superficial division
are from retina and visual cortex, additional afferents may also
exist. For example, Astruc (1971) demonstrated sparse degeneration
in SGS and SO after lesions in area 8 (arcuate sulcus), though
Kuypers and Lawrence (1967) report degeneration only in SO after
similar lesions. In the cat a fiber projection from auditory area
AII has been shown to terminate in SGS (Paula-Barbosa et al.,
1973), but a similar projection from the homologous area of monkey
cortex was not reported by Whitlock and Nauta (1956).

Afferents to the Deep Division. In the deep division of the
SC are located those premotor neurons which most convincingly
suggest that this structure plays a role in the control of eye
movements (see below). It is also in this region that an amazing
number of fiber systems arising from both non-visual and visually
related structures from virtually all levels of the CNS converge.
These are briefly described below.

The deep division receives afferents from many cortical areas
(Astruc, 1971; Hirasawa, 1938; Kuypers and Lawrence, 1967; Mettler,
1935; Myers, 1963; Petras, 1971; Thompson, 1900; Whitlock and
Nauta, 1956). Among these areas are the frontal pole, arcuate
sulcus (area 8), ventral portions of the precentral gyrus and
rostral pericentral gyrus, a very light projection from postcentral
gyrus and caudal pericentral gyrus with the projection heaviest
from the ventral third of these regions, some fibers from the
inferior parietal lobule terminating in a caudal area of deep SC
and heavy projections from temporal lobe and occipital lobe
(Kuypers and Lawrence, 1967). The temporal lobe projection has
been studied in some detail by Whitlock and Nauta (1956). Fibers
projecting to the deep division were found throughout the temporal
lobe except from anterior regions of the inferior temporal sulcus.
Auditory koniocortex was not lesioned in their experiment. The
anterior temporal pole terminates in the lateral one third, medial
temporal sulcus in the lateral half, caudal inferior temporal
sulcus in the anterior two thirds of the deep division. A lesion
confined to the middle of the superior temporal sulcus terminated
in the posteriolateral colliculus. Recently, Ogren and Hendrickson
(1976) reported a similar projection from superior temporal
sulcus in squirrel monkey. Petras (1971) has suggested that the
parietomesencephalic fibers might permit tactile and proprioceptive
information to be distributed to mesencephalic visual areas which
are concerned with visually guided behavior. At the present time
we can only speculate on the frame of reference for the topographical
projection to colliculus from some cortical regions.

The subcortical afferents to the deep division have been
given little attention in monkey from an anatomical standpoint,
the literature being more detailed in the cat. In monkey, inputs
have been demonstrated from the inferior colliculus (Barnes et
al., 1943 (in monkey); Moore and Goldberg, 1963; Powell and Hatton,
1969 in cat), the ventral portion of the posterior commissure and
interstitial nucleus of Cajal (Carpenter et al., 1970) and portions
of Gower's tract (spinotectal; (Poirier and Bertrand, 1955).
Substantia nigra projects bilaterally (Carpenter and McMasters,
1964) and the sublentiform nucleus (a pretectal nucleus) projects
ipsilaterally to the deep division (Santos-Anderson et al., 1976).
Other subcortical afferents probably also exist. In cat, for
example, fastigiotectal (Angaut 1969; Thomas et al., 1956) and
periaqueductal grey (Hamilton, 1976) projections have been described
and homologous systems will probably be found in monkey.

Efferent Projections of the SC

The efferent projections of the SC can at present be divided
into three major groupings, the ascending efferents from the
superficial division, the ascending efferents from the deep division

and the descending efferents from the deep division. The ascending
projections provide a means by which visual (superficial) and
multimodal and movement-related (deep) information processed in
the SC can be disseminated to thalamocortical systems (feedback?)
while the descending projection is distributed to premotor systems
in the brainstem. The efferent projections of many of the thalamic
targets of the SC have been discussed recently (Benevento and
Rezak, 1975; Burton and Jones, 1976) and will not be presented
here.

       Ascending Projections. The ascending projections of the SC
have been described with degeneration methods by Benevento and
Fallon (1975) and to a lesser extent by Myers (1963 and personal
communication). The superficial division sends fibers to the
dorsal LGN[1] (magnocellular layers), ventral LGN and the inferior
pulvinar (particularly the medial portion) via the brachium of the
SC. Fibers also project, via the medial pretectum, to the anterior
pretectal nucleus and pretectal region. Sparse degeneration was
also found in the dorsomedial nucleus and centrointermediate
nucleus. After more anterior lesions in the superficial layers
additional sparse degeneration was found in the limitans nucleus,
some intralaminar nuclei and the lateral posterior nucleus. These
additional thalamic relay sites of the anterior SC (central visual
field), though possibly due to damage of fibers en passage (Benevento
and Fallon, 1975), are not unexpected in view of the varying
density of retinotectal and corticotectal fibers to posterior and
anterior SC. Pericellular degeneration resulting from superficial
lesions was found in the ipsilateral colliculus within 0.75mm of
the lesion and no degeneration was reported in the contralateral
colliculus.

       Projection sites of the deep layers were found in the medial
pulvinar and, to a lesser extent, oral pulvinar, the central gray,
medial geniculate nucleus, suprageniculate nucleus, limitans
nucleus, nucleus of the accessory optic tract, zona incerta, all
intralaminar nuclei, dorsomedial nuclei, olivary nucleus, reuniens
nucleus and dorsomedial nuclei. The projections to thalamic
nuclei appeared to be topographic -- deep and superficial anterior
colliculus to posterior thalamic nuclei and deep and superficial
posterior SC to anterior areas of the same thalamic nuclei (Benevento
and Fallon, 1975).

       Descending Projections. Descending efferents from the deep
division have been described autoradiographically by Harting
(1976). Fibers leave the deep layers in two major tracts, the

_____
[1]A similar projection from SC to dorsal LGN has been described
in grey squirrel (Robson and Hall, 1976) and in cat (Nimi, et al.,
1970).

crossed predorsal bundle and the ipsilateral tectopontine and
tectobulbar tracts. Predorsal bundle terminations can be found
predominantly in the contralateral nucleus reticularis pontis
oralis and caudalis. Dense terminations also occurred ventral to
the abducens nucleus, with some label found in the rostral portion
of this nucleus. The ipsilateral projection of the deep layers is
to the parabigeminal nucleus, mesencephalic reticular formation,
the dorsal lateral pontine gray and, minimally, in the nucleus
reticularis tegmenti pontis, cuneiform nucleus, nucleus reticularis
pontis caudalis, the external nucleus of the inferior colliculus,
the substantia nigra, and, via the intertectal commissure, the
contralateral SC. There appears to be no SC fibers which terminate
in the cerebellum (Truex and Carpenter, 1971 p. 424). While
several of the terminal regions of these descending fibers may be
indirectly related to oculomotor function, other terminations
(ventral abducens area, pontine nuclear regions along the midline)
have been clearly implicated in oculomotor processing (Keller,
1974; Highstein et al., 1976).

Intracollicular Organization

Fibers enter and leave the SC from both the superficial and
deep divisions. It is, therefore, necessary to ask how information
is processed within and between these divisions. Unfortunately,
there is almost a total lack of data, both in terms of anatomy and
electrophysiology, relevant to this point in the monkey. Keeping
this in mind, the following discussion depends for the most part
on Golgi studies in the mouse, rat, cat and hedgehog (Cajal, 1954;
Langer, 1971; Langer and Lund, 1974; Sterling, 1971; Tokunaga,
1970; Tokunaga and Otani, 1976; Valverde, 1973; Victorov, 1966,
1968).

Within each division there appears to be considerable neuronal
interaction. The dendritic fields of most cells in the SC are
distributed either within the lamina containing the soma or into
the adjacent lamina. Within each division, there are intrinsic
axons which terminate in the division of origin, e.g. marginal
cells have intrinsic axons with an extensive local distribution.
Based on the frequency of horizontal cell processes, it would
appear that lateral processing within each division is considerable,
particularly in the SGS, but to a lesser extent in the deeper
layers (e.g. superficial and deep horizontal cells).

Although, as Sprague (1975) has suggested, each lamina may
have a "certain independence" from other lamina, there are significant interconnections between lamina. For example, the cylindrical
neurons of Tokunaga and Otani (1976) have axons which course in a
ventralward direction and are likely to terminate within the SC.
Other intrinsic axons have also been observed to ascend towards
the SO from more ventral tiers.

LESION OR ABLATION STUDIES

Effects Noted by Gross Examination of Eye Movements

Contradictory results are reported following SC ablation in the monkey. Denny-Brown and Fischer (1976) observed one monkey with total, bilateral removal of the SC with some pretectal and periaqueductal involvement. This animal was completely unresponsive to visual stimuli except for blink responses to bright light. Conjugate eye movements in all directions could be evoked by tactile stimuli. Other monkeys with less complete removal of the colliculus (with some infringement of the inferior colliculus) were initially inactive, mute, "staring aimlessly into space" although they explored for food when hungry. They made reaching movements, unaccompanied by visual fixation to large moving objects. Postoperative recovery was first noted for the optokinetic response followed by recovery of visual placing responses and, later, vision for moving objects. Localization of stationary objects was the last visual function to show recovery (Denny-Brown, 1962).

Pasik, Pasik and Bender (1966) observed the effects of SC lesions upon spontaneous gaze, pursuit movements, oculomotor responses to tactile and auditory stimuli, oculocephalic reflexes and optokinetic and vestibular nystagmus. They report that "none of our observations on conjugate gaze deviations, whether spontaneous or pursuit, those associated with lid closure or with turning of the head, optically or vestibularly induced, and the ocular responses to auditory or somesthetic stimuli revealed an enduring deficit after almost total ablation of both superior colliculi."

The reasons for the differences in the findings of these two studies are not apparent since lesions and survival times were comparable. It should be emphasized that both studies based their conclusions on gross examination of eye movements. In neither study was the ability of the animal to foveate a visual stimulus examined.

Anderson and Symmes (1968) studied 13 monkeys with bilateral lesions of the SC. Lesions were incomplete with considerable sparing of the anterior regions of the colliculus. During the early postoperative period animals exhibited, with varying severity, some or all of the following signs: "apparent blindness, visual agnosia, failure to follow objects moved through one or either visual field, fixed gaze, lethargy and areflexia, and disequilibrium." These effects were not persistent and subsequently, eye movements in all directions with "normal amplitude and briskness" were observed. Monkeys undisturbed in their home cages, however, displayed fewer exploratory and food searching eye movements than normal animals. Formal testing revealed that discrimination of rate of movement was severely impaired in animals with bilateral collicular damage. On the other hand, longer lasting symptoms of fixed gaze (Cardu et al., 1975; Rosvold et al., 1958) and absence of coordinated eye movements (Cardu et al., 1975) have been reported.

Effects on Accuracy of Reaching

Indirect evidence for the role of the SC in the control of eye movements may be derived from studies reporting deficits in the accuracy of reaching responses following collicular lesions. Keating (1974) tested the ability of monkeys with bilateral collicular lesions to reach to the location of the dimmer of two briefly (200 msec) flashed spots of light. Lesioned monkeys required from 1-10 times the number of preoperative errors to regain criterion. The pattern of errors suggested that performance was poorest for stimuli falling in the peripheral visual field. Since in this experiment, the stimulus and response panels were large (approximately 15 deg in diameter), the head was unrestrained and there was no control of fixation, error magnitude could not be determined but must have been large. Keating noted that monkeys with tectal lesions showed a "reluctance" to make large angular eye movements. The deficit in the accuracy of reaching movements was confirmed by Keating (1976) in an experiment examining the effects of SC ablations combined with lesions of the macular retina. The retinal lesions forced the monkeys to solve the reaching task with peripheral vision but the effects of tectal lesions were not exaggerated.

Butter (1974) produced small to moderately large bilateral SC lesions in rhesus monkeys. These lesions frequently spared the ventral layers, the most lateral and the anterior and posterior extremes of the SC. Monkeys were tested for retention of a pattern discrimination task and for the acquisition of a color discrimination. The monkey's task was to displace one of two stimulus plaques covering two food wells. The plaques could be displaced only by pushing at one edge of the stimulus plaque (the response site). The discriminative stimulus (present throughout the trial) was located at the response site on some trials and displaced from the response site on others. Lesioned animals showed deficits only when stimuli were displaced from the response site. Butter suggested that the deficit in performance may reflect a reduced ability of animals with collicular lesions to produce alternating fixation of the stimulus and response loci.

MacKinnon et al. (1976) trained monkeys to reach to a specific site indicated by a small light of 5 sec duration to obtain a raisin. The visual cue was directly in front of the food compartment and the light was extinguished before animals were allowed to respond. After tectal lesions monkeys continued to perform the task normally, but showed a severe deficit if the visual cue was reduced to 1 sec duration.

Studies Using Direct Measurements of Eye Movement

The effects of SC lesions upon the accuracy and latency of
eye movements has been measured directly in monkeys trained on a
saccadic tracking task. Wurtz and Goldberg (1972) tested the
effects of relatively small and of larger unilateral lesions upon
accuracy and latency of visually-elicited saccades. Both small
and large lesions produced an increase of 150-300 msec in the
latency of a saccade to a stimulus in the region of the visual
field projecting to the lesioned area. No deficit in the accuracy
of the saccades and only a transient change in the velocity of eye
movements were observed. Transient effects observed after large
lesions included a paucity of spontaneous eye movements to the
contralateral side and deviation of eye position to the side of
the lesion.

The finding that the accuracy of saccades is unaffected by
collicular lesions may need to be modified in light of several
recent but brief reports. Collicular lesions can produce inaccurate
saccades (Schiller, 1972) a higher frequency of double saccades to
acquire a visual target (Wurtz and Mohler, 1976) and deficiencies
in foveating peripheral stimuli (Kurtz and Butter, 1976). Detailed
reports of these experiments are not available, however.

Comparative Considerations

The lesion data for the monkey should be considered in the
context of studies using other mammals as subjects. Schneider
(1969) demonstrated that undercutting the SC of the golden hamster
abolishes the ability of the animal to orient toward an object but
not the ability to identify it. In the tree shrew (Tupaia glis)
a similar failure to orient to moving food stimuli following
removal of the deep layers of the SC has been observed (Casagrande
and Diamond, 1974; Raczkowski et al., 1976). Such animals are
able to avoid obstacles and to orient toward and approach doorways
in a barrier test. They are capable of learning some types of
visual discriminations (vertical vs. horizontal stripes or red vs.
blue), but not others. These animals appear blind when in their
home cage and fail to follow or orient to food objects or to avoid
threatening objects. A similar deficit does not accompany lesions
involving only the superficial gray and optic layers.

Thus, lesions of the SC in other mammals produce dramatic and
long-lasting deficits in the ability to orient to visual and
auditory stimuli. In the rhesus monkey, the deficits are less
severe and recovery is more rapid.

Comment and Directions for Further Study

Lesion studies which used only gross observations of eye movements found that saccadic movements can and do occur in monkeys in which the SC has been almost totally removed. From these studies it appears that although severe postoperative effects may be observed and longer lasting deficits in latency and accuracy occur, the SC is not an essential structure for saccade occurrence. However, when refined measurements of eye movements are used the saccades which do occur are slower and inaccurate, requiring multiple saccades to acquire visual targets. Furthermore, the frequency of spontaneous movements is reduced and animals show some symptoms of visual field neglect.

The finding that the SC is not an essential structure for saccade occurrence should not be surprising, perhaps. In a complex visual environment, the oculomotor system is capable of generating saccades to acquire visual targets based upon shape, size, hue or other properties of the visual stimulus. It is unlikely that exactly the same subset of visual and oculomotor neurons are involved in each of these tasks. In visually-elicited saccades, the oculomotor system draws upon the analytical power of various visual "channels" (depending upon the contingencies of the current tracking task) to compute the spatial coordinates of the target. A single lesion is unlikely to incapacitate the system since most tasks can be solved using alternative strategies and other computational elements. Thus, animals with lesions of the visual cortex (Mohler and Wurtz, 1974), the frontal eye fields (Latto and Cowey, 1971) and the SC are, upon recovery, capable of producing saccades and fixations of visual targets. This point of view is consistent with recent reports (Mohler and Wurtz, 1974) of accurate visual tracking after removal of the visual cortex, but not after removal of both visual cortex and SC. To date, permanent deficits in the ability to generate saccades are observed only following destruction of premotor neurons synaptically close to the final common pathway or following actual destruction of motor neurons (Hoyt and Daroff, 1971).

It is also important to note that the effects of SC lesions upon the accuracy of eye movements have been assessed using limited behavioral tasks, such as tracking the movement of a single dot in an otherwise blank field. Even in these experiments, the details of the movements (such as velocity, number of corrective saccades, and magnitude of error) have not been examined closely. The accuracy of movements requiring integration of several modalities (for example, the accuracy of eye movements when the position of the head is varied) has not been determined. Nor has the ability of the monkey with collicular lesions to select one of several simultaneously presented stimuli been investigated. What are the

effects of SC lesions upon the ability of the oculomotor system to
make predictive saccadic movements such as those occurring during
visual search or to make saccades to a stimulus, the location of
which is stored in memory?

Recent demonstrations of temporary recalibration of the
saccadic system (Matin, 1972; Pola, 1974) suggest that malleable
neural mechanisms are involved in programming saccade amplitude
and direction. Is the SC which receives inputs from a variety of
peripheral and central areas, involved in the process of recalibration? Are animals with SC lesions capable of reorganizing
visuo-oculomotor functions following prolonged exposure to inverting
lenses? What are the effects of SC lesions made during early
development upon the subsequent development of oculomotor functions?

STIMULATION STUDIES

Early Experiments

Adamuk (1872) first reported that electrical stimulation of
the SC produced conjugate eye movements. Evoked movements resembled
those of normal animals and the direction of movements was dependent
upon the site of stimulation within the colliculus. Stimulation
medially produced up and lateral movements; stimulation laterally
produced down and lateral movements.

Hess and coworkers (1946) found that electrical stimulation
of the SC of chronically prepared cats produced conjugate movements
of the eyes and head. They proposed that the colliculus was
responsible for a "visual grasp reflex" which brings about fixation
of moving objects.

Apter (1946) discovered that after small crystals of powdered
strychnine sulfate were placed on specific regions of the colliculus
of lightly anesthetized cats, diffuse photic stimulation resulted
in movements whose directions and amplitudes were dependent upon
the site of the crystal placement. When discrete retinal stimulation
was used, the occurrence of eye movement was dependent upon
stimulation of regions of the retina which projected to the region
of the SC where the crystal had been placed. Based upon these
results, Apter, in an early statement of the foveation hypothesis,
stated:

"The superior colliculus is, therefore, one station in the
reflex pathway which mediates movements of both eyes toward a
light flash in the peripheral visual field. It also appears
from the data that the systematic arrangement of retinal
fibers on the superior colliculus has a motor counterpart;

that is, particular areas on the colliculus are responsible
for conjugate movement of the eyes toward the particular
place in the visual field projecting to the area on the
colliculus."

Experiments Using Monkeys as Subjects

Robinson (1972) extended Apter's findings in the cat by
stimulating the SC of alert monkeys and by using a sensitive
magnetic search coil to measure horizontal and vertical eye
positions. Stimulation with constant current pulse trains (500/sec;
0.5 sec duration) produced contralateral saccades whose amplitude
and direction were dependent upon the site of stimulation within
the colliculus. Vergence, smooth, nystagmic or disconjugate
movements were never observed. Within broad limits, the evoked
movements were independent of stimulus parameters and of the
location of the eye in the orbit. Across the colliculus, the
saccades were small (1 deg) anteriorly, large (50 deg) posteriorly
and had up components medially, down components laterally. An
extensive map of the amplitude and direction of elicited saccades
was developed and this motor map was found to overlap the sensory
map formed by the retinotectal projection to the superficial
layers of the SC.

Threshold currents required to evoke saccades varied as a
function of depth in the colliculus. Thresholds were as high as
800 uA near the surface of the colliculus, remained at about 200
uA for 1-1.5 mm through the intermediate layers and then abruptly
dropped to around 20 uA as electrodes entered the deep layers.
Latencies of movements produced by superficial stimulation were
typically 30 msec and never shorter than the 20 msec latencies
observed following stimulation of the deep layers.

Schiller and Stryker (1972) confirmed the stimulation results
of Robinson in experiments with monkeys in which microelectrodes
were used for both recording and stimulation. In the superficial
layers, neurons were activated by stimuli from a particular region
of the visual field. Stimulation produced saccades which allowed
this region of visual space to project to the fovea. In the
deeper layers, neuronal activity preceded spontaneously occurring
saccades with specific amplitudes and directions and stimulation
produced similar movements.

The SC does not appear to be involved in the initiation of
head movements. Collicular stimulation in monkeys free to move
their heads in the horizontal plane produced short latency, repeatable
eye movements with definite thresholds (Stryker and Schiller,
1975). Direction and amplitude of evoked saccades were independent
of initial eye position. In contrast, evoked head movements were

variable in size and latency, did not have definite electrical
thresholds, and were dependent upon initial eye position. Head
movements were most likely to follow stimulation when the eyes
were in a position of extreme deviation. The conclusion that the
monkey SC is not directly involved in the initiation of head
movements is also supported by the failure of Robinson and Jarvis
(1974) to find SC unit activity uniquely related to head movements.

Experiments Using Cats as Subjects

Stimulation of the anterior SC produces saccades with particular
directions and amplitudes which are independent of initial eye
position (see Roucoux and Crommelinck, 1976 for references). As
in the monkey, the motor map produced by stimulation is similar to
the sensory map formed by the retinotectal projection to the SC.
Saccades evoked by repeated stimulation of a collicular point are
more variable in the cat than in the monkey. This is not surprising,
since the cat does not have a fovea, as such, and a wider range of
eye movements would be effective in bringing a target to the
relatively large area centralis.

However, stimulation of the posterior SC in the cat (with
the head restrained) evokes goal-directed movements; that is, the
eyes reach the same final position in the orbit when the colliculus
is stimulated, regardless of initial eye position. The most
eccentric final positions are observed upon stimulation of the
most posterior SC; stimulation medially produces up final positions,
and lateral stimulation produces down final positions (Roucoux and
Crommelinck, 1976).

In the cat, pinnae movements are also evoked by stimulation
of the SC (Schaefer, 1970). The direction of pinnae movements is
related to electrode position. Stimulation of anterior sites
produces forward turning of both pinnae, stimulation of middle
sites produce forward turning of the ipsilateral pinna and, sometimes,
backward orientation of the contralateral pinna. (Schiller,
personal communication, sometimes observed pinnae movements in the
monkey following stimulation of the posterior SC but this has not
been extensively investigated).

Comment and Directions for Further Study

Movements elicited by stimulation of any point in the monkey
SC or by stimulation of the anterior portion of the cat colliculus
have a retinal frame of reference. Both animals act as if a
specific region of the retina were being activated and, accordingly,
eye movements are independent of the position of the eye in the
orbit. In contrast, the frame of reference of movements elicited
by stimulation of the posterior SC of the cat is, perhaps, the

head. Upon stimulation of the posterior SC, the cat acts as if a
stimulus occurred at a specific location in the environment and
saccades move the eye toward the location regardless of initial
eye position. The neuronal mechanisms by which retinal error
signals, neck and extra ocular muscle afferent signals, and perhaps
efference copy and other signals are integrated to permit "goal-
directed" movements are not understood.

Investigations examining the latency and other characteristics
of eye movements evoked by microstimulation of brain regions
receiving efferent projections from the SC should provide useful
information. Determination of the latency of the evoked saccades
and of the current required for evoking the movements should
indicate whether the stimulated brain area is synaptically closer
than the SC to motor neurons. Evoked movements may be qualitatively
different from those produced by SC stimulation. If so, results
could provide important clues concerning the signal transformations
which occur subsequent to the colliculus.

ELECTROPHYSIOLOGICAL STUDIES

Response to Visual Stimuli

The responses of SC neurons to visual stimuli have been
studied in both anesthetized (Cyander and Berman, 1972) and alert
monkeys (Goldberg and Wurtz, 1972; Schiller and Koerner, 1971;
Schiller and Stryker, 1972). Despite differing methodologies and
schemes for classifying neuronal responses, there is considerable
agreement concerning the response of SC neurons to visual stimuli.
The receptive field organization is described below.

The Superficial Layers (SGS and SO)

Receptive field properties. All the neurons encountered in
the superficial layers are visually responsive. Most units respond
to the onset of a stationary spot of light with a phasic on-
response, and to the termination of the stimulus with an off-
response. A tonic discharge is recorded from some SC neurons
during the stimulus presentation. Most units are binocularly
driven and have circular or ellipsoidal responsive areas with
suppressive or inhibitory surrounds. A gradient of response
intensity may occur across the excitatory area of the receptive
field, with weaker responses occurring near the edges of the
field.

Receptive field size varies as a function of eccentricity in
the visual field. Diameters as small as 0.75 deg were observed
for units responsive to stimulation of the macular region whereas

neurons responsive to peripheral stimulation can have receptive
field diameters of 20-30 deg or larger. As successive units are
encountered in an electrode penetration perpendicular to the
surface of the colliculus, cells with the smallest receptive
fields are encountered first and receptive field diameters increase
with depth.

Topographical Organization of Receptive Fields. The visual
field is mapped, topographically, upon the superficial layers of
the SC. The perifoveal representation is enlarged with over one
third of the collicular surface devoted to the central 10 deg of
the visual field. Cells in the superficial layers of each colliculus
are activated by stimuli in the contralateral visual half-field.
Neurons with receptive fields in the upper visual field are located
medially; those with receptive fields in the lower visual field
are located laterally. Units with receptive fields near the
center of the visual field are located anterioraly, those with
receptive fields in the periphery are located posteriorly. The
representation of the horizontal meridian runs from anteriolateral
to posteriomedial.

Shape Sensitivity. Cells in the SC are not shape sensitive.
Cells respond equally well to small circles, annuli, ellipsoids,
or to stimuli with concave, convex, serrated or straight edges.

Contrast Sensitivity. Cynader and Berman (1972) report that
neurons in the superficial layers of the colliculus repond equally
well to dark or light objects. Updyke (1974) found 7% of the
units preferred light edges, 41% preferred dark edges and the
remainder responded equally well to light or dark edges entering
the excitatory field.

Size Sensitivity. According to Updyke (1974) some neurons
are not differentially sensitive to stimulus size unless the
boundaries of the excitatory region are exceeded, some respond
best to stimuli filling the excitatory region of the receptive
field and some respond best to stimuli smaller than the excitatory
region. Schiller and Koerner (1972) report that the optimal
stimulus diameter seldom exceeds 5 deg of visual angle. Goldberg
and Wurtz (1972) failed to find spatial summation in the receptive
field but Updyke (1974) reports both spatial summation and spatial
suppression.

Movement Sensitivity. Neurons in the superficial layers
respond best to stimuli moving 0.5 to 30 deg/sec although some
cells continue to respond to stimulus velocities as high as 800
deg/sec. Only 10% of the cells in the superficial layers are
directionally selective, and these cells are broadly tuned. An
orderly arrangement of directionally selective/cells in the
colliculus, as found in the cat, has not been observed in the monkey.

Orientation Sensitivity. Most neurons in the superficial layers do not exhibit orientation specificity although the optimal stimulus for directionally selective neurons is an edge oriented perpendicular to the optimal direction of movement.

Object Specificity. Updyke[1] (1974) found some units which gave maximal responses upon presentation of three-dimensional objects in their receptive fields. Some units in the lower half of the SGS and SO responded exclusively to objects.

Color Specificity. Neurons in the SC are characterized as broad-band and not color-opponent cells (Marrocco and Li, 1976; Malpeli and Schiller, 1976).

Intermediate Layers (SGI and SAI)

The receptive fields of visually responsive neurons in the intermediate layers are larger than those of neurons found in the superficial layers. Receptive fields are circular, ellipsoidal or even rectangular in shape and range from 1 to 70 degrees in diameter. Neurons are not shape or orientation selective and have low spontaneous activity levels. "Newness" or "novelty" neurons which respond best to suddenly appearing stimuli are seen in the intermediate layers. Many cells in this layer show rapid habituation.

Deep Layers (SGP and SAP)

Visually responsive neurons isolated in the deeper layers of the SC have larger receptive fields than neurons lying above them in more superficial layers, are binocularly driven, and many respond to stimuli of other modalities, including tactile and auditory stimuli. Auditory stimuli which failed to elicit a neural response were capable of enhancing the response to visual stimuli (Cynader and Berman, 1972). Cells found in this layer exhibited a prolonged afterdischarge (lasting as long as 10 sec.) when novel stimuli were presented.

Updyke (1974) reports that half of all the deeper-layer cells he encountered were sensitive to object stimuli. Of these, some responded optimally to objects approaching or held in close proximity to the animal's head. Two of these units responded to either auditory or visual stimuli approaching the animal.

---

[1]Updyke used Cebus monkeys and this may account for some differences between this observation and those of other researchers.

Response to Non-Visual Stimuli

The non-visual afferents to the SC have not received careful attention in the monkey, although auditory and tactile responses have been observed (Updyke, 1974; Wurtz and Goldberg, 1972).

In the cat, the SC receives proprioceptive (from limb, neck, and extrinsic eye muscles) (Abrahams and Rose, 1975), auditory and somatosensory (see Stein et al., 1976 for references) as well as visual inputs. The superficial layers are thought to be exclusively visual whereas neurons responsive to visual or non-visual stimuli (or both) are encountered in the deeper laminae. Bimodal and trimodal neurons have been observed in the intermediate and deeper layers of the SC.

Gordon (1973) found that if a cell in the SC of the cat responded to both auditory and visual stimuli, the auditory and visual receptive fields were overlapping (both auditory and visual stimuli were effective only when moving through a particular region of space). Stein et al., (1976) observed a stratified organization of visual, somatic and acoustic modalities within the cat SC. The magnified representation of central visual fields overlapped the magnified tactile representation of the face and, as visual receptive fields moved temporally in the visual field, the underlying tactile receptive fields were displaced posteriorly and distally on the body surface. A similar arrangement was observed in the mouse (Dräger and Hubel, 1975, 1976).

Abrahams and Rose (1975) report projections to the SC of the cat from fore and hindlimb muscle nerves as well as from neck and oculomotor muscle afferents. Most units activated by limb afferent nerve stimulation also respond to visual stimuli and many of the cells excited by these afferents are cells of origin of the tectospinal pathway.

The visual, auditory and tactile neurons isolated in the intermediate and deeper layers all have large receptive fields and habituate rapidly. For each modality there are both peripheral and cortical inputs and these terminate in comparable regions of the colliculus (see anatomy section). The multimodality neurons are located in the same region of the colliculus in which movement-related activity is isolated in chronic experiments, but it is not known whether or not the multimodality and movement-related responses originate from the same or different neurons.

Relationship of Neuronal Activity in the Superior
Colliculus to Eye Movements

General properties of movement fields. Chronic microelectrode
recording techniques have shown that the maximal discharge of
neurons in the deeper layers of the monkey SC occurs prior to an
eye movement with a particular direction and amplitude (Robinson
and Jarvis, 1971; Schiller and Koerner, 1971; Schiller and Stryker,
1972; Sparks, 1975; Sparks, Holland and Guthrie, 1976; Wurtz and
Goldberg, 1972).   These neurons have a movement field, i.e., the
neuron discharges prior to a range of movements of similar directions
and amplitudes. Unit discharge occurs (for different neurons)
from 10-150 msec prior to saccades and is independent of the
initial position of the eye in the orbit. Furthermore, some of
these neurons discharge prior to movements in total darkness and
prior to the quick phases of optokinetic and caloric nystagmus.

A gradient of response magnitude is observed across the
movement fields. A vigorous discharge precedes movements to the
center of the movement field, but reduced responses precede movements
which deviate from this direction and/or amplitude. Movement
field size is a function of the amplitude of the optical movement.
Neurons discharging prior to small saccades have small and sharply
tuned fields. Neurons discharging prior to large saccades have
large movement fields and tuning is relatively coarse (Sparks et
al., 1976).

Movement fields of SC neurons may also be characterized by a
temporal gradient. The interval between the onset of spike discharge
and the onset of a saccade is greater for movements near the
center of the movement field than for movements to the periphery
of the field (Sparks et al., 1976).

There are at least two, and probably more, categories of SC
neurons with saccade-related activity. Some neurons which discharge
prior to saccades also have visual receptive fields, other neurons
have only movement fields. Neurons which discharge in response to
visual stimuli and prior to eye movements have overlapping, but
not necessarily co-extensive movement and receptive fields.

Topographical Distribution of Movement-related Neurons. Movement fields are topographically organized within the SC with
neurons discharging prior to small saccades located anteriorly and
neurons firing before large saccades located posteriorly. Cells
near the midline discharge prior to movements with up components
and cells laterally discharge maximally before movements with down
components.

Mohler and Wurtz (1976) recently reported that during most
electrode penetrations of the SC, the interval between spike

discharge and saccade onset is less for the first movement-related
neuron encountered within the intermediate layers than for neurons
encountered subsequently during the penetration. They conclude,
accordingly, that the cells located in the more superficial regions
of the intermediate layer cannot be providing the only input to
the cells deeper in this layer. They also reported the isolation
of neurons at the border of the superficial and intermediate
layers which discharged before visually triggered saccades, but
not before spontaneously occurring saccades of similar amplitudes
and directions.

    Coupling Between Spike Activity and Saccade Occurrence. If
the SC is involved in the initiation of saccades then one might
expect to isolate a subpopulation of these neurons in which the
onset of the neuronal response is tightly coupled to saccade
onset. Furthermore, in a situation in which the occurrence of a
visual stimulus sometimes elicits a saccade and sometimes fails to
do so, the probability of a neural response should be highly
correlated with the probability of saccade occurrence.

    Mohler and Wurtz (1976) isolated fifteen cells in which the
neuronal burst could be dissociated from the occurrence of eye
movements. In a situation in which a visual target was presented
for only 100-200 msec the monkey sometimes made a saccade to the
target and sometimes did not. A neural discharge sometimes occurred
both when the monkey failed to make a saccade to acquire the
target or when the target was acquired by two saccades (not normally
associated with a discharge) instead of one. When the target was
repeatedly presented at the same position, allowing the animal to
predict target location, the neural discharge sometimes preceded
target onset. Thus, Mohler and Wurtz argue that the discharge of
movement cells is more closely related to the monkey's readiness
to make an eye movement than to the execution of the eye movement
itself.

    We have recently completed a similar experiment in which the
coupling between movement-related neuronal activity and saccade
occurrence was examined. We also studied the relationship between
the latency of the behavioral response and the latency of the
neural response. The experimental design is outlined in Figure 1.

    We isolated one type of SC neuron which generates a pulse of
spike activity beginning approximately 20 msec before the onset of
saccades with particular amplitudes and directions (see Figure 2).
These neurons did not give a visual response, only a movement-
related response. For this type neuron, there was a high degree
of relationship between the occurrence of the pulse of spike
activity and the occurrence of the saccade associated with this
activity.

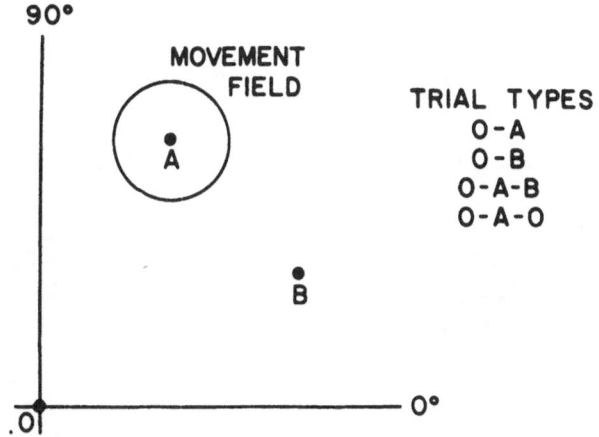

FIGURE 1. The tracking task. Four types of trials were presented
randomly. During O-A trials, monkeys were required to fixate
a target at the center of the screen (O) and after a variable
interval the target was moved to a position near the center
of the movement field of the neuron (A). If the animal
acquired the target within 400 msec and maintained fixation
for 2 sec., a liquid reward was presented. During O-B trials,
after a variable duration of fixation of point O, the target
was moved to point B. Saccades to acquire B were not in the
movement field of the neuron being investigated. O-A-B and
O-A-O trials required an initial fixation of point O. Then,
the target was moved to A for a chosen interval, T_1. At the
end of the interval, the target was moved to B (or O) and remained there until acquired by the subject. At particular
durations of T_1, a saccade was made to A and then a second
saccade was made to B (or O). On other trials, with the same
T_1 interval, the saccade to A did not occur and either the
monkey maintained fixation of O (O-A-O) or a single saccade
to B occurred (O-A-B).

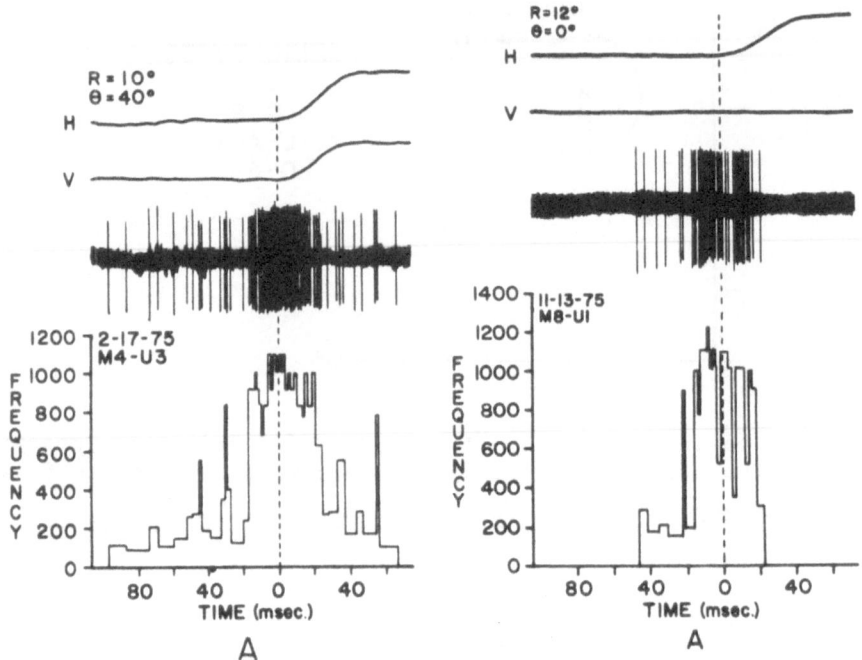

FIGURE 2. Discharge patterns recorded from two movement-related
neurons in the superior colliculus. H: horizontal eye position.
V: vertical eye position. Middle tracing: spike activity.
Bottom graph: instantaneous spike frequency. The dotted line
represents the onset of the eye movement. Examination of the
instantaneous frequency record reveals that for both neurons,
there is a relatively discrete pulse of spike activity occurring
approximately 20 msec prior to saccade onset.

Figure 3 illustrates typical experimental results for this type neuron. On those trials in which an appropriate saccade occurred, the neural activity which precedes the saccade is composed of two parts - a prepulse build-up of activity followed by a fairly discrete pulse of activity. On those trials in which an appropriate saccade did not occur, only the prepulse activity was observed.

Figure 4 shows, for one neuron, the least vigorous burst associated with a movement to the center of its movement field and the most vigorous burst which occurred on those trials in which a saccade to the movement field did not occur. The neural responses occurring in the absence of a saccade to the movement field would appear as vigorous bursts of activity when displayed as rasters with the resolution used by Mohler and Wurtz (1976). However, when the spike activity is viewed with greater resolution, there is a clear distinction between the most vigorous responses occurring in the absence of a saccade and the least vigorous responses occurring prior to an appropriate saccade.

For these neurons, the pulse of spike activity was tightly coupled to saccade onset. This is illustrated in Figure 5. Spike pulse and saccade latencies were measured for 38 saccades to the same point in the movement field for the neuron illustrated on the left and for 50 saccades for the neuron illustrated on the right. The high degree of association is apparent.

When different cells were compared, burst duration was not correlated with optimal saccade amplitude. Burst duration of neurons firing maximally to 3 deg saccades was as great as (or greater than) burst duration of neurons firing maximally to 10 deg movements. Nor was cell discharge specifically correlated with either the vertical or horizontal components of associated saccades. This is in contrast to what was observed in the burst neurons of the pontine reticular formation (Keller, 1974; Luschei and Fuchs, 1972; Sparks and Travis, 1971).

Although these are correlational data and do not permit cause and effect statements to be made, we feel that these data support the foveation hypothesis of SC function. There is a response of SC neurons which is tightly coupled to the onset of appropriate saccades and the probability of occurrence of this response is highly correlated with the probability of saccade occurrence.

Properties of Afferent Signals to the Superior Colliculus

Retinal Afferents. The SC receives input from both concentric and nonconcentric broad-band retinal ganglion cells, but not from

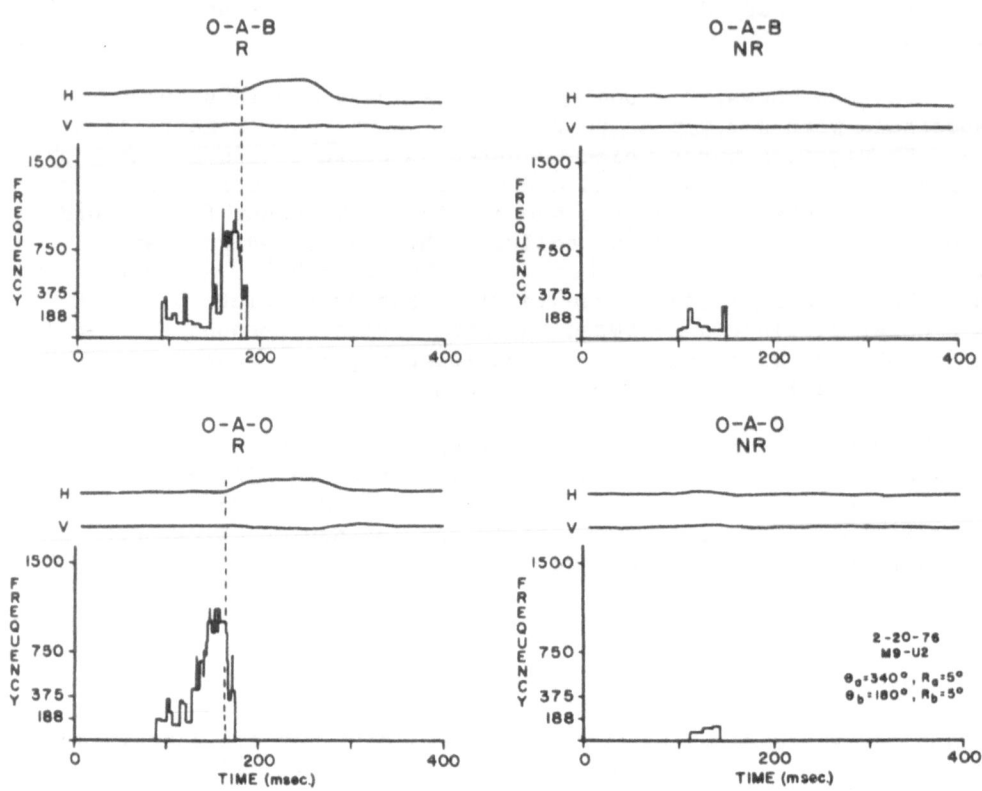

FIGURE 3. Top left: O-A-B trial with a saccade to A and a second
     saccade to acquire B. In the instantaneous frequency record,
     there is some prepulse activity followed by a discrete pulse
     of activity. Top right: O-A-B trial with a single saccade
     to acquire B. Some build-up of spike activity is seen, but
     a pulse of activity was not present. Bottom left: O-A-O
     trials with a saccade to O and a saccade to reacquire O. A
     discrete pulse of spike activity occurred. Bottom right:
     O-A-O trial in which the monkey maintained fixation of O.
     Some build-up of spike activity was observed, but a discrete
     pulse of activity was not present.

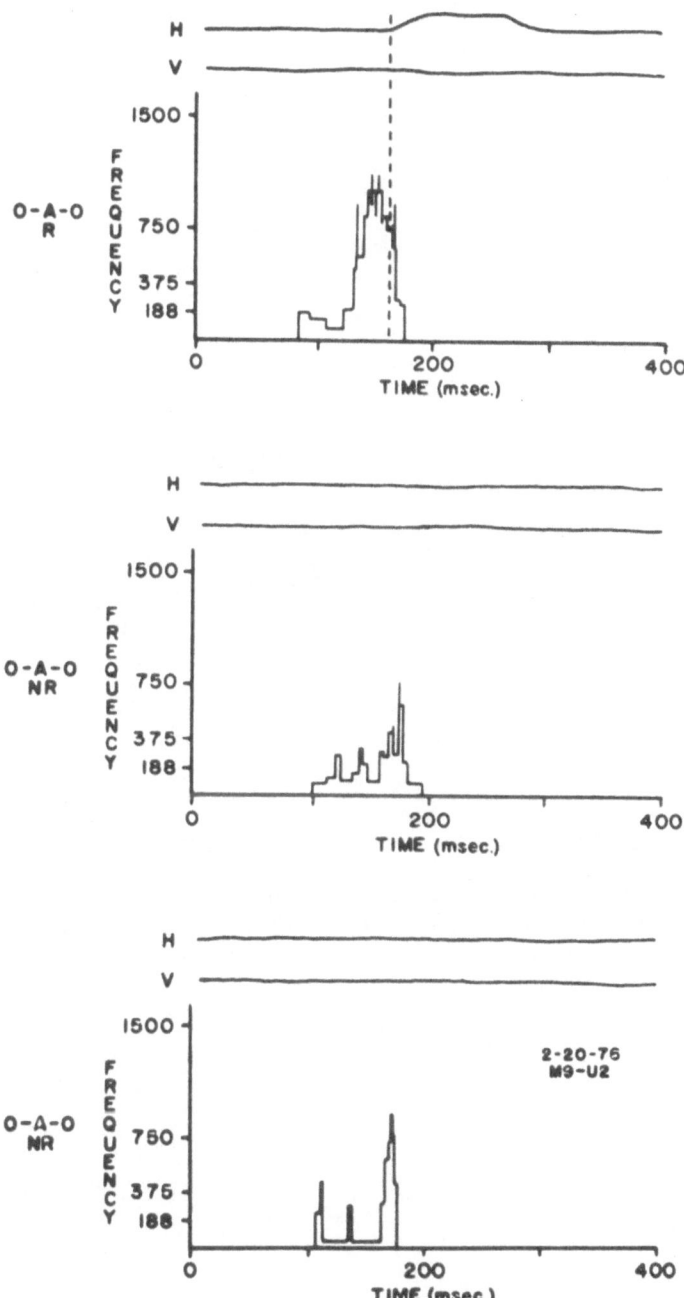

FIGURE 4. Top: least vigorous burst associated with a movement to the center of the movement field for one neuron. Middle and bottom: most vigorous burst on O–A–O trials in which a response to A did not occur.

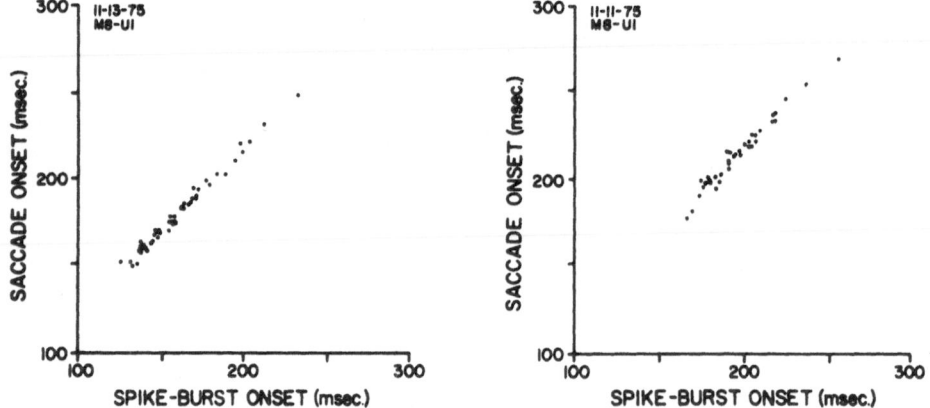

FIGURE 5. Relationship between spike burst latency and saccade
    latency for two neurons. The abscissa represents the interval
    between target onset and the onset of the spike pulse. The
    ordinate represents saccade latency.

color-opponent cells (Malpeli and Schiller, 1976; de Monasterio, 1976). The major retinal input is from cells with nonconcentric receptive fields which have slowly conducting axons, low spontaneous activity and broad-band color sensitivity.

Inputs from visual cortex. Lund et al. (1975) used the retrograde transport of horseradish peroxidase to identify efferent cells of area 17 of the monkey. The projection to the SC arises from pyramidal neurons of all sizes lying in lamina 5B. Finlay, Schiller and Volman (1975) have shown that it is the cortical cells with complex receptive field properties which project to the SC. Of the cells in the visual cortex, the corticotectal cells have the largest receptive fields and have the least preferences for orientation. Twenty percent of the corticotectal neurons are orientation specific and only 30% are directionally-selective.

The receptive field properties of cells in the SGS and in the dorsal part of the SO are largely unaffected by ablation of the visual cortex (Schiller et al., 1974). Some cells, however, do not respond uniformly to visual stimuli throughout their receptive fields and there are subtle changes in the ocular dominance distribution following visual cortex ablation. In the deeper layers of the SC, visual responses can no longer be elicited after visual cortex ablation. Similarly, cortical cooling has little or no effect on the response of neurons in the superficial layers but disrupts visual responses below this region. Eye movement cells in the deeper layers of the SC of the alert monkey are still present after ablation of the visual cortex, but they no longer have visual receptive fields.

Other Inputs. Neurons responding to visual stimuli (Mohler et al., 1973) and neurons discharging after saccades (Bizzi, 1968; Bizzi and Schiller, 1970; Mohler et al., 1973) have been isolated in the frontal cortex. The frontal eye fields are known to project to the SC but the properties of the frontal lobe corticotectal cells have not been determined. Similarly, the parietal cortex is known to project to the SC (Kuypers and Lawrence, 1967; Petras, 1971) and neurons in this area have been isolated which respond to visual stimuli. Other neurons discharge prior to saccades to acquire motivationally significant stimuli (Mountcastle et al., 1975). Which, if any, of these neuron types project to the colliculus is unknown.

Experiments are needed similar to those of Finlay et al. (1975) in which the corticotectal neurons are identified by antidromic responses to collicular stimulation. Then their functional properties can be determined and compared to the response properties of collicular neurons. Similar studies are needed to determine the properties of the inputs arriving to the colliculus from other cortical and subcortical areas as well.

Collicular Influences on Motoneurons

The linkage of the SC to motor neurons of the extra-ocular muscles has not been examined in the monkey. Intracellular recordings in the cat by Precht et al. (1974) indicate that the tecto-abducens linkage is polysynaptic with a possible disynaptic connection. Grantyn and Grantyn (1976), also in the cat, found evidence of a major disynaptic pathway from colliculus to the abducens nucleus. They noted that approximately one quarter of the reticular neurons ventral and rostroventral to the abducens were monosynaptically activated by SC stimulation. Procion yellow injections into some of these reticular neurons showed axonal projections to or through the abducens nucleus. Some axons traversed the abducens and entered the medial longitudinal fasciculus.

Comment and Directions for Further Study

Despite the recent surge of interest in SC function, many questions remain unanswered. We have outlined below three directions for future research which, in our opinion, are particularly important.

What Role Do Auditory and Somatosensory Inputs Play In Superior Colliculus Function? The function of auditory and somatosensory inputs to the SC may not be directly related to the initiation of saccadic eye movements. For example, these signals could function to modify visual activity originating from a specific region of the environment. On the other hand, SC neurons responding to auditory and somatosensory stimuli may provide information concerning the source of a stimulus and participate in the initiation of orienting eye movements. Do SC neurons discharge prior to saccades elicited by auditory or tactile stimuli? If so (considering only the auditory input), at least two possibilities exist: auditory and visual inputs may converge upon the same movement-related neurons, or a separate population of movement-related neurons, receiving primarily auditory inputs, may exist. If auditory and visual inputs converge upon the same set of movement-related neurons, is the head the frame of reference for the auditory inputs? If so, how are the differences between the foveal (visual) and head (auditory) frame of references resolved? If separate populations exist for saccades elicited by auditory stimuli, what is the frame of reference for these neurons?

We have recently undertaken equipment modifications which will allow us to train monkeys to track auditory as well as visual stimuli. We hope to provide answers to some of these questions in experiments soon to be under way.

Target Selection. An important issue, which has received relatively little attention is the question of how, in a complex

visual environment, particular stimuli are chosen as targets for
foveal acquisition. Since only a small region of the visual field
can be viewed foveally, some mechanism must exist for selecting
this region.

Neurons with large receptive fields, many of which respond to
more than one modality input and which show the property of rapid
habituation, are found in the intermediate and deeper layers of
the SC. The convergence of central inputs and of peripheral
stimuli from several modalities provides a mechanism by which
spatially or temporally contiguous novel stimuli could alter the
responsiveness of visual and/or movement-related neurons. The
simultaneous occurrence of an auditory and a visual stimulus in
one region of the environment could produce (through spatial
summation) an enhanced response of neurons in a specific region of
the topographically organized SC. Similarly, these neurons could
alter the probability that particular movement-related neurons
would be activated. (This, of course, presumes that the spatial
location of auditory, visual, and somatosensory inputs are kept in
some type of alignment.)

The cortical inputs to SC provide a circuit by which a
particular stimulus may be "stored" until a saccade to acquire the
stimulus is generated. Close examination of the activity of neurons
in the superficial layers sometimes reveals a repetitive discharge
at approximately 70 msec intervals, which continues until a saccade
occurs or until a decision to acquire another target is made.
This pattern of activity is particularly noticeable on trials with
brief targets in which the animal seems to be postponing a saccade
in order to see whether or not the stimulus will move or remain in
that location. This may be an important function since the response
of most SC neurons to a steady stimulus is a brief transient on-
reponse. Thus, the position of stimuli which are viewed by the
organism as potential targets for foveal viewing may be periodically
refreshed in the SC. Other stimuli produce a single, transient
on-response.

At the present time there is little data which can be used to
argue for or against these speculations. The intrinsic connections
of the SC are poorly understood and the speculations cannot be
supported or rejected on anatomical grounds. The effects of
auditory or tactile stimuli upon the visual responsiveness of
either the visual neurons in the superficial layers or the movement-
related neurons in the deeper layers is unknown. Goldberg and
Wurtz (1972) and Wurtz and Mohler (1976) have observed an enhancement
of the response of cells in the superficial layers of the SC to
visual stimuli when those stimuli are used as targets for saccades.
The enhancement is spatially and temporally limited and does not
occur if the stimulus is a target for a hand, rather than an eye,

movement. The enhanced response to stimuli in one region of the
visual field is not accompanied by depressed responsiveness to
stimuli in other areas of the visual field. Enhancement of the
response of visual neurons in the dorsal layers of the SC may be
one mechanism by which selectivity occurs.

Once a target has been selected, is there a mechanism for
preventing the occurrence of competing movements? Suppose that
neurons discharging prior to saccades reduce the sensitivity of
sensory and other movement neurons. Such an inhibition prior to
and during saccadic movements would function to clear the visual
register, thereby resetting the foveal frame of reference for the
retino-topic coordinates of the SC. The collateral suppression of
movement neurons would prevent other saccades from changing the
course of the impending movement.

We have preliminary data which suggest that the responsiveness
of visual neurons in the superficial layers is markedly suppressed
slightly before and during saccades. The neural response to a
stimulus in the receptive field failed to occur if presented 20-30
msec. prior to a saccade to acquire a stimulus out of the receptive
field. We have not yet determined the temporal or spatial extent
of these effects nor do we have control data indicating that this
is not a backward masking effect due to visual rather than efferent
influences.

How Can Neurons With Large Receptive and Movement Fields
Generate Precise Saccades? One argument against the foveation
hypothesis is that the receptive and movement fields of SC neurons
are too large to direct precise movements. In an attempt to
assess the validity of this argument, we measured the response
gradient across the movement fields of SC neurons and found that
the gradient was not sharply tuned to specific movements, particularly
for neurons discharging prior to saccades larger than 5 deg in
amplitude (Sparks et al., 1976). Since a single movement-related
neuron discharges prior to a wide range of saccades, a large
region of the SC will be active prior to a specific saccade (we
were unable to determine the exact distribution of this activity).
We concluded that precise information about saccade direction and
amplitude (if present in the colliculus) must be encoded in the
collective discharge of a large number of cells since the discharge
of any one movement cell is ambiguous as to the exact saccade
direction and amplitude.

We presented a simple model (Sparks et al., 1976) similar to
the one proposed to McIlwain (1975) by which precise saccades can
be initiated by SC neurons with large movement fields. According
to this model, saccade direction and amplitude are determined by
the spatial location of the population of neurons active in the

intermediate and deeper layers of the SC. The precision or accuracy
of a saccade results from the summation of the movement tendencies
produced by the population of neurons rather than the discharge of
a small number of finely tuned neurons. The contribution of each
neuron to the direction and amplitude of the movement is relatively
small. Consequently, the effects of variability or noise in the
discharge frequency of a particular neuron are reduced by averaging
over many neurons. One line of future research planned in our
laboratory is a test of this model of SC function.

CONCLUSION

The SC is a complex structure with multiple inputs and
outputs and probably has multiple functions. Clearly, as the
review of anatomical, stimulation, electrophysiological, and
lesion data indicates, one of these functions is concerned with
the initiation of saccadic eye movements.

Current data, in our opinion, is compatible with the view
that the SC functions to trigger, under a certain set of conditions,
eye movements with particular amplitudes and directions. The
direction and amplitude of saccades are coded spatially within the
SC. Each saccade is preceded by neuronal activity from a population
of neurons located in a specific region of the SC. It is the
location of the neurons in the SC and not the pattern of spike
activity originating from the neurons which encodes saccade amplitude
and direction. The spike discharge of the neuron only functions
to trigger an appropriate output. The generation of efferent
signals appropriate for each of the extraocular muscles is an
intrinsic property of the subsequent pattern of activity triggered
by SC neurons.

The neuronal circuitry which accepts the SC trigger and
generates the actual pattern of motor neuron activity necessary to
produce specific movements has not yet been described.

ACKNOWLEDGEMENTS

We thank Drs. Peter Schiller, Terry Hickey and Larry Mays for
valuable criticism of an early version of this paper. We thank
Dick Holland for technical assistance and Sally Marcus for assistance
in preparing the manuscript.

This work was supported by NIH Grant EY01189. Jay G. Pollack was
supported by a NEI Postdoctoral Research Fellowship 1 F32EY05112.

REFERENCES

Abrahams, V. C. and Rose, P. K. Projections of extraocular, neck
    muscle and retinal afferents to superior colliculus in the
    cat: Their connections to cells of origin of tectospinal
    tract. *J. Neurophysiol.*, 38:10–18, 1975.

Adamuk, E. Über angeborene and erworbene association. von F. C.
    Donders. *v. Graefes Arch. Ophthal.*, 18;153–164, 1972.

Anderson, K. V., and Symmes, D. The superior colliculus and
    higher visual functions in the monkey. *Brain Res.*, 13:37–52,
    1969.

Angaut, P. The fastigio-tectal projections: An anatomical experi-
    mental study. *Brain Res.*, 13:186–189, 1969.

Apter, J. T. Eye movements following strychninization of the
    superior colliculus of cats. *J. Neurophysiol.*, 9:73–86,
    1946.

Astruc, J. Corticofugal connections of area 9 (frontal eye field)
    in <u>Macaca</u> <u>mulatta</u>. *Brain Res.*, 33:241–256, 1971.

Barnes, W. T., Magoun, H. W. and Ranson, S. W. The ascending
    auditory pathway in the brain stem of the monkey. *J. Comp.
    Neurol.* 79: 129–152, 1943.

Benevento, L. A. and Fallon, J. H. The ascending projections of
    the superior colliculus in the rhesus monkey. *J. Comp.
    Neurol.*, 169: 339–362, 1975.

Benevento, L. A., and Rezak, M. The cortical projections of the
    inferior pulvinar and adjacent lateral pulvinar in the rhesus
    monkey <u>(Macaca</u> <u>mulatta</u>): An autoradiographic study. *Brain
    Res.*, 108:1–24, 1976.

Bizzi, E. Discharge of frontal eye field neurons during saccadic
    and following eye movements in unanesthetized monkeys. *Exp.
    Brain Res.*, 10:69–80, 1968.

Bizzi, E. and Schiller, P. H. Single unit activity in the frontal
    eye fields of unanesthetized monkeys during eye and head
    movement. *Exp. Brain Res.*, 10:151–158, 1970.

Black, P. and Myers, R. E. Connections of occipital lobe in
    monkey. *Anat. Rec.*, 142:216–216, 1962.

Bunt, A. H., Hendrickson, A. E., Lund, J. S., Lund, R. D., and Fuchs, A. F. Monkey retinal ganglion cells: Morphometric analysis and tracing of axonal projections, with a consideration of the peroxidase technique. *J. Comp. Neurol.*, 164:265-286, 1975.

Burton, H. and Jones, E. G. The posterior thalamic region and its cortical projection in new world and old world monkeys. *J. Comp. Neurol.*, 168:249-302, 1976.

Butter, C. M. Effects of superior colliculus, striate, and prestriate lesions on visual sampling in Rhesus monkeys. *J. Comp. Physiol.* Psychol., 87:905-917, 1974.

Cajal, S. R. Histologie du systeme nerveux de l'homme et des vértebrés. II. Maloine, Paris, 1954.

Campos-Ortega, J. A. and Hayhow, W. R. On the organization of the visual cortical projection to the pulvinar in Macaca mulatta. *Brain Behav. Evol.*, 6:394-423, 1972.

Cardu, B., Ptito, M., Dumont, M., and Lepore, E. Effects of ablations of the superior colliculi on spectral sensitivity in monkeys. *Neuropsychol.*, 13:297-306, 1975.

Carpenter, M. B., Harbison, J. W., and Peter, P. Accessory oculomotor nuclei in the monkey: Projections and effects of discrete lesions. *J. Comp. Neurol.*, 140:131-153, 1970.

Carpenter, M. B., and McMasters, R. E. Lesions of the substantia nigra in the rhesus monkey: Efferent fiber degeneration and behavioral observations. *Amer. J. Anat.*, 114:293-312, 1964.

Casagrande, V. A., Harting, J. J., Hall, W. C. and Diamond, I. T. Superior colliculus of the Tree Shrew: A structural and functional subdivision into superficial and deep layers. *Science*, 177: 444-447, 1972.

Casagrande, V. A. and Diamond, I. T. Ablation study of the superior colliculus in the tree shrew (Tupaia glis). *J. Comp. Neurol.* 156:207-238, 1974.

Cynader, M. and Berman, N. Receptive field organization of monkey superior colliculus. *J. Neurophysiol.*, 35:187-219, 1972.

Denny-Brown, D. and Fischer, E. G. Physiological aspects of visual perception. II. The subcortical visual direction of behavior. *Arch. Neurol.*, 33:228-242, 1976.

Denny-Brown, D. The midbrain and motor integration. *Proc. Roy Soc. Med.*, 55:527-538, 1962.

Dräger, U. C. and Hubel, D. H. Responses to visual stimulation and relationship between visual, auditory, and somatosensory inputs in mouse superior colliculus. *J. Neurophysiol.*, 38:690-713, 1975.

Dräger, U. C. and Hubel, D. H. Topography of visual and somatosensory projections to mouse superior colliculus. *J. Neurophysiol.*, 39:91-101, 1976.

Finlay, B. L., Schiller, P. H., and Volman, S. F. The receptive field properties of corticotectal cells in striate cortex of the Rhesus monkey. Personal Communication.

Garey, L. J., Jones, E. G., and Powell, T. P. S. Interrelationships of striate and extrastriate cortex with the primary relay sites of the visual pathway. *J. Neurol. Neurosurg. Psychiat.*, 31:135-157, 1968.

Gilbert, D. C. and Kelly, J. P. The projections of cells in different layers of the cat's visual cortex. *J. Comp. Neurol.*, 163:81-106, 1975.

Goldberg, M. E., and Wurtz, R. H. Activity of superior colliculus in behaving monkey. I. Visual receptive fields of single neurons. *J. Neurophysiol.*, 35:542-559, 1972.

Gordon, B. Receptive fields in deep layers of cat superior colliculus. *J. Neurophysiol.*, 36:157-178, 1973.

Grantyn, A. A. and Grantyn, R. Synaptic actions of tectofugal pathways on abducens motoneurons in the cat. *Brain Res.*, 105:269-285, 1976.

Graybiel, A. M. Evidence for banding of the cat's ipsilateral retinotectal connection. *Brain Res.*, 114:318-327, 1976.

Hamilton, B. L. Projections of the nuclei of the periaqueductal gray matter of the cat. *J. Comp. Neurol.*, 152:45-58, 1974.

Harting, J. K. Descending pathways from the monkey superior colliculus. *Soc. Neurosci. 6th Ann. Meet.*, abstract, 1976.

Harting, J. K., Hall, W. C., Diamond, I. T., and Martin, G. F. Anterograde degeneration study of the superior colliculus in Tupaia glis: Evidence for a subdivision between superficial and deep layers. *J. Comp. Neurol.*, 148:361-386, 1973.

Hendrickson, A., Wilson, M. E., and Toyne, M. L. The distribution of optic nerve fibers in Macaca mulatta. *Brain Res.*, 23:425-427, 1970.

Hess, W. R., Burgi, S., and Bucher, V. Motorische Funktion des Tektal-und Tegmental-gebietes. *Monats. Psychiatr. Neurol.*, 112:1-52, 1946.

Highstein, S. M., Mackawa, K., Steinacker, A., and Cohen, B. Synaptic input from the pontine reticular nuclei to abducens motoneurons and internuclear neurons in the cat. *Brain Res.*, 112:162-167, 1976.

Hirasawa, K., Okano, S. and Kamio, S. Beitrag zur kenntnis über die corticalen extra-pyramidalen fäsern aus der area temporalis superior (area 22) beim affen. *Z. Mikr. Anat. Forsch.*, 44:74-84, 1938.

Hoyt, W. F. and Daroff, R. M. Supranuclear disorders of ocular control systems in man. In: *The Control of Eye Movements.* ed. Bach-y-Rita and Collins, C. C., Academic Press, N.Y.:175-235, 1971.

Hubel, D. H., LeVay, S. and Wiesel, T. M. Mode of termination of retinotectal fibers in macaque monkey; an autoradiographic study. *Brain Res.*, 96:25-40, 1975.

Ingle, D. and Sprague, J. M. (Eds) Sensorimotor Function of the midbrain tectum. *Neurosci. Res. Prog. Bull.*, Vol. 13, No. 2 1975.

Keating, E. G. Impaired orientation after primate tectal lesions. *Brain Res.*, 67:538-541, 1974.

Keating, E. G. Effects of tectal lesions on peripheral field vision in the monkey. *Brain Res.*, 104:316-320, 1976.

Keller, E. L. Participation of medial pontine reticular formation in eye movement generation in monkey. *J. Neurophysiol.*, 37:316-331, 1974.

Kurtz, D., and Butter, C. M. Deficits in visual discrimination performance and eye movements following superior colliculus ablations in rhesus monkeys. *Soc. Neurosci. 6th Ann. Meet.*, abstract, 1976.

Kuypers, H. G. J. M., and Lawrence, D. G. Cortical projections to the red nucleus and the brain stem in the rhesus monkey. *Brain Res.*, 4:151-188, 1967.

Langer, T., and Lund, R. D.   The upper layers of the superior
    colliculus of the rat.   A Golgi study.   *J. Comp. Neurol.*,
    158:405-436, 1974.

Langer, T.   Cellular patterns in the superior colliculus of the
    rat.   A Golgi study.   Masters thesis.   U. Wash., Seattle,
    Washington 1971.

Latto, R. and Cowey, A.   Fixation changes after frontal eye-field
    lesions in monkeys.   *Brain Res.*, 30:25-36, 1971.

Lund, J. S., Lund, R. D., Hendrickson, A. E., Bunt, A. H. and
    Fuchs, A. F.   The origin of efferent pathways from the primary
    visual cortex, area 17, of the macaque monkey as shown by
    retrograde transport of horseradish peroxidase.   *J. Comp
    Neurol.*, 164:287-304, 1975.

Lund, J. S. and Boothe, R. G.   Interlaminar connections and
    pyramidal neuron organization in the visual cortex, area 17,
    of the macaque monkey.   *J. Comp. Neurol.*, 159:305-334, 1975.

Lund, R. D.   Terminal distribution in the superior colliculus of
    fibers originating in the visual cortex.   *Nature*, 204:1283-
    1285, 1964.

Lund, R. D.   Synaptic patterns in the superficial layers of the
    superior colliculus of the monkey, Macaca mulatta.   *Exp.
    Brain Res.*, 15:194-211, 1972.

Luschei, E. S. and Fuchs, A. F.   Activity of brain stem neurons
    during eye movements of alert monkeys.   *J. Neurophysiol.*,
    35:445-461, 1972.

MacKinnon, D. A., Gross, C. G., and Bender, D. G.   A visual
    deficit after superior colliculus lesions in monkeys.   *Acta.
    Neurobiol. Exp.*, 36: 169-180, 1976.

Magalhaes-Castro, H. H., Murata, L. A., and Magalhaes-Castro, B.
    Cat retinal ganglion cells projecting to the superior colliculus
    as shown by the horseradish peroxidase method.   *Exp. Brain
    Res.*, 25:541-549, 1976.

Malpeli, J. G. and Schiller, P. H.   Properties of monkey retinal
    ganglion cells and their tectal projections.   *Soc. Neurosci.
    6th Ann. Meet.*, abstract, 1976.

Mandl, G.   The influence of visual pattern combinations on responses
    of movement sensitive cells in the cat's superior colliculus.
    Brain Res., 75:215-240, 1974.

Marrocco, R. T. and Li, R.   Retinotectal input to monkey superior colliculus. *Soc. Neurosci. 6th Ann. Meet.*, abstract, 1976.

Matin, L.   Eye movements and perceived visual direction.   In: *Handbook of Sensory Physiology*.   Vol. VII/4 Visual psychophysics.   ed. Jameson, D. and Hurvich, L. M.   Springer-Verlag, N.Y.: Pp. 331–380, 1972.

McIlwain, J. T.   Visual receptive fields and their images in superior colliculus of the cat. *J. Neurophysiol.*, 38:219–230, 1975.

Mettler, F. A.   Corticofugal fiber connections of the cortex of Macaca mulatta.   The parietal region. *J. Comp. Neurol.*, 62:263–291, 1935.

Mohler, C. W., Goldberg, M. E. and Wurtz, R. H.   Visual receptive fields of frontal eye field neurons. *Brain Res.*, 61:385–389, 1973.

Mohler, C. W. and Wurtz, R. N.   Organization of monkey superior colliculus; intermediate layer cells discharging before eye movements. *J. Neurophysiol.*, 39:722–744, 1976.

Mohler, C. W. and Wurtz, R. H.   Role of striate cortex and superior colliculus in visual guidance of saccadic eye movements in monkey. *Soc. Neurosci. 4th Ann. Meet.*, abstract, 1974.

de Monasterio, S. M.   Properties of linear and non-linear ganglion cells in monkey retina. Personal Communication.

Moore, R. Y. and Goldberg, J. M.   Ascending projections of the inferior colliculus in the cat. *J. Comp. Neurol.*, 121:109–136, 1963.

Mountcastle, V. B., Lynch, J. C., Georgopoulos, A., Sakata, H., and Acuna, C.   Posterior parietal association cortex of the monkey: Command functions for operations within extrapersonal space. *J. Neurophysiol.*, 38:871–908, 1975.

Myers, R. E.   Striate cortex connections in the monkey. *Fed. Proc.*, 21:352, 1962.

Myers, R. E.   Cortical projections to midbrain in monkey. *Anat. Rec.* 145:337–338, 1963.

Nimi, K., Miki, M. and Kawamura, S.   Ascending projections of the superior colliculus in the cat. *Okjimas Folia Anat. Jap.*, 269–287, 1970.

Ogren, M. and Hendrickson, A.   Connections between extrastriate
    cortex and thalamus in squirrel monkey.   *Soc. Neurosci. 6th
    Ann. Meet.*, abstract, 1976.

Palmer, L. A., Rosenquist, A. C., and Sprague, J. M.   Cortico-
    tectal systems in the cat: Their structure and function.
    In: *Corticothalamic Projections and Sensorimotor Activities.*
    eds. Frigyesi, T. L., Rinvik, E., and Yahr, M. D., Raven
    Press: N.Y., pp. 491-522, 1972.

Pasik, T., Pasik, P., and Bender, M. B.   The superior colliculus
    and eye movements.   *Arch. Neurol.*, 15:420-436, 1966.

Paula-Barbosa, M. M. and Sousa-Pinto, A.   Auditory cortical
    projections to the superior colliculus in the cat.   *Brain
    Res.*, 50:47-61, 1973.

Petras, J. M.   Connections of the parietal lobe.   *J. Psychiat.
    Res.*, 8:189-201, 1971.

Poirier, L. J. and Bertrand, C.   Experimental and anatomical
    investigation of the lateral spino-thalamic and spinotectal
    tracts.   *J. Comp. Neurol.*, 102:745-758, 1955.

Pola, J.   The relation of the perception of visual direction to
    eye position during and following a voluntary saccade.
    Unpublished doctoral dissertation, Columbia University, 1974.

Powell, E. W., and Hatton, J. B.   Projections of the inferior
    colliculus in the cat.   *J. Comp. Neurol.*, 136:183-192, 1969.

Precht, W., Schwindt, P. C. and Magherini, P. C.   Tectal influences
    on cat ocular motoneurons.   *Brain Res.*, 82: 27-40, 1974.

Raczkowski, D., Casagrande, V. A., Diamond, I. T.   Visual neglect
    in the Tree Shrew after interruption of the descending
    projections of the deep superior colliculus.   *Exp. Neurol.*,
    50:14-29, 1976.

Robinson, D. A.   Eye movements evoked by collicular stimulation in
    the alert monkey.   *Vision Res.*, 12:1795-1808, 1972.

Robinson, D. L. and Jarvis, D. C.   Neurons of single units in
    superior colliculus of the alert rhesus monkey.   *J. Neuro-
    physiol.*, 34:925-936, 1971.

Robson, J. A. and Hall, W. C.   Projections from the superior
    colliculus to the dorsal lateral geniculate nucleus of the
    grey squirrel (Sciurus carolinensis).   *Brain Res.*, 113:379-
    385, 1976.

Rosvold, H. E., Mishkin, M. and Szwarcbart, M. K. Effects of subcortical lesions in monkeys on visual discrimination and single alternation performance. *J. Comp. Physiol. Psychol.*, 51:437–444, 1958.

Roucoux, A. and Crommelinck, M. Eye movements evoked by superior colliculus stimulation in the alert cat. *Brain Res.*, 106:349–363, 1976.

Santos-Anderson, R., Rezak, M., and Benevento, L. A. An autoradiographic study of the projections of the pretectum in the macaque monkey. *Soc. Neurosci. 6th Ann. Meet.*, abstract, 1976.

Schaefer, K. P. Unit analysis and electrical stimulation in the optic tectum of rabbits and cats. *Brain Behav. Evol.*, 3:222–240, 1970.

Schiller, P. H. Some functional characteristics of the superior colliculus of the rhesus monkey. In: *Cerebral Control of Eye Movements and Motion Perception*, ed. Dichgans, J., and Bizzi, E. Basel: S. Karger, pp. 122–129, 1972.

Schiller, P. H. and Koerner, F. Discharge characteristics of single units in superior colliculus of the alert rhesus monkey. *J. Neurophysiol.*, 34:920–924, 1971.

Schiller, P. H., Stryker, M., Cynader, M., and Berman, N. Response characteristics of single cells in the monkey superior colliculus following ablation or cooling of visual cortex. *J. Neurophysiol.*, 37:181–194, 1974.

Schiller, P. H. and Stryker, M. Single-unit recording and stimulation in superior colliculus of the alert rhesus monkey. *J. Neurophysiol.*, 35:915–924, 1972.

Schneider, G. E. Two visual systems. *Science*, 163:895–902, 1969.

Sparks, D. L., and Travis, R. P., Jr., Firing patterns of reticular formation neurons during horizontal eye movements. *Brain Res.*, 90:147–152, 1975.

Sparks, D. L., Holland, R. and Guthrie, B. L. Size and distribution of movement fields in the monkey superior colliculus. *Brain Res.*, 113:21–34, 1976.

Sprague, J. M. Mammalian Tectum: intrinsic organization, afferent inputs, and integrative mechanism. In: *Sensorimotor Function of the Midbrain Tectum*. ed. Ingle, D., and Sprague, J. M. *NRP Bull.*, 13:204–213, 1975.

Sprague, J. M., Berlucchi, G., and Rizzolatti, G. The role of the
    superior colliculus and pretectum in vision and visually
    guided behavior. In: R. Jung (Ed.), *Handbook of Sensory
    Physiology*. Vol. VII/3 Central processing of visual information.
    Part B. Visual centers in the brain. Springer-Verlag: N.Y.,
    pp. 27-101, 1973.

Stein, B. E., Magalhaes-Castro, B. and Kruger, L. Relationship
    between visual and tactile representation in cat superior
    colliculus. *J. Neurophysiol.*, 39:401-419, 1976.

Sterling, P. Receptive fields and synaptic organization of the
    superficial gray layer of the cat superior colliculus.
    Vision Res. Suppl., 3:309-328, 1971.

Stryker, M. P. and Schiller, P. H. Eye and head movements evoked
    by electrical stimulation of monkey superior colliculus.
    Exp. Brain Res., 23:103-112, 1975.

Thomas, D. M., Kaufman, D. P., Sprague, J. M., and Chambers, W. N.
    Experimental studies of the vermal cerebellar projections in
    the brain stem of the cat (fastigio-bulbar tract). *J.
    Anat. Lond.*, 90:371-385, 1956.

Thompson, W. H. Degenerations resulting from lesions of the
    cortex of the temporal lobe. *J. Anat. Physiol.*, 35:147-165,
    1900.

Tokunaga, A. Neuronal structure of the superior colliculus of the
    rat. *Chiba Igakkai Zasshi*, 46:298-299, 1970.

Tokunaga, A. and Otani, K. Dendritic patterns of neurons in the
    rat superior colliculus. *Exp. Neurol.*, 52:189-205, 1976.

Truex, R. C. and Carpenter, M. B. *Human Neuroanatomy*, Williams
    and Wilkins Co: Baltimore, Maryland, 1969.

Updyke, B. V. Characteristics of unit responses in superior
    colliculus of the cebus monkey. *J. Neurophysiol.*, 37:896-
    909, 1974.

Valverde, F. The neuropil in superficial layers of the superior
    colliculus of the mouse. *Z. Anat. Entwicki.-Gesch.*, 142:117-
    147, 1973.

Victorov, I. V. Neuronal structure of the superior colliculus in
    the cat. *Arch. Anat.*, 2:45-55, 1968.

Victorov, I. V. Neuronal structure of the anterior corpora bigemina in Insectivora and rodents. *Arkh. Anat. Gistol. Empriol.*, 8: 82–89, 1966.

Walls, G. L. *The Vertebrate Eye and its Adaptive Radiation*, Hafner Publishing Co.: New York, 1967.

Wilson, M. E. and Toyne, M. J. Retinotectal and corticotectal projections in Macaca mulatta. *Brain Res.*, 24:395–406, 1970.

Wurtz, R. H. and Goldberg, M. E. Activity of superior colliclus in behaving monkey. III. Cells discharging before eye movement. *J. Neurophysiol.*, 35:575–586, 1972.

Wurtz, R. H. and Goldberg, M. E. Activity of superior colliculus in behaving monkey. IV. Effects of lesions on eye movement. *J. Neurophysiol.*, 35:587–596, 1972.

Wurtz, R. H. and Mohler, C. W. Organization of monkey superior colliculus; Enhanced visual response of superficial layer cells. *J. Neurophysiol.*, 89:745–764, 1976.

INDEX

Abducens nerve palsy, 72
Abducens nucleus, 127 et. seq.
   antidromic response, 128,
      131 et. seq.
   EPSPs, 133 et. seq.
   H^3-proline studies, 135
   horseradish peroxidase
      studies, 128
   IPSPs, 133 et. seq.
   orthodromic response, 131,
      132, et. seq.
Basal ganglia, 53
Cerebellum, 65 et. seq.
   climbing fibers, 67, 69, 79
   complex spikes, 77
   flocculus and nodulus, 67, 75
   mossy fibers, 67, 69, 75, 80
   parallel T fibers, 67, 70, 79
   projections to brainstem, 151
   simple spikes, 77
   and vestibulo-ocular reflex,
      65 et. seq.
Cervico-ocular reflex, 24, 28, 33
Coding, vector, 116
Congenital ocular motor apraxia,
   5, 52
   optokinetic nystagmus, 20
   saccadic eye movements, 19,
      20, 52
   vestibulo-ocular reflex, 23, 53
   head dysmetria, 20
Control system - continuous, 42
Control system - discrete, 42
Dysmetria, 17, 19, 45, 67, 72
   vestibulo-ocular reflex, 66, 68
Eighth nerve, 68

Eye-head coordination, 9 et.
   seq., 66
   brain stem, 16
   cerebellum, 16
   predictable mode, 16
   superior colliculus, 16
   supranuclear control, 16
   triggered mode, 10, 16
   vestibular system, 16, 19,
      24, 33, 52
Gegenrücken, 45, 53
Glissade, 46
Horseradish peroxidase
   in abducens nucleus, 121, 128
   in oculomotor nucleus, 121
   in vestibulo-cerebellar
      pathway, 150 et. seq.
Inferior olive, 67, 69, 77
Internuclear ophthalmoplegia,
   45, 54, 59, 72, 127
Macro square wave jerks, 45,
   53, 59
Medial longitudinal fasciculus,
   45, 52, 108, 127 et. seq.
   constituent neurones, 139
   and gaze paresis, 127
   and inter-nuclear ophthal-
      moplegia, 127
   path to medial rectus,
      127 et. seq.
   stimulation of, 135
Medial rectus, 127 et. seq.
Myasthenia gravis, 3, 4
Nucleus gigantocellularis, 105
Nucleus intercalatus of
      Stadverini, 145 et. seq.

Nucleus of Roller, 145 et. seq.
Nucleus prepositus hypoglossi,
    145 et. seq.
  and cerebellum, 168 et. seq.
  and reticular formation, 167
    et. seq.
  and superior colliculus, 170
    et. seq.
  and vestibular system, 167
    et. seq.
  burst tonic units, 167 et. seq.
  directional selectivity of
    units, 169
  EPSPs, 156
  eye position, 165
  IPSPs, 156
  optokinetic nystagmus, 163
  projection to trochlear moto-
    neurons, 161 et. seq.
  tonic units, 167 et. seq.
  vestibular nystagmus, 163
  nucleus reticularis pontis
    caudalis (n.r.p.c.), 105,133
    et. seq.
  nucleus reticularis pontis
    oralis (n.r.p.o.), 105, 133
    et. seq.
Nystagmus, 54, 68
  caloric-induced, 52
  congenital, 1, 2, 45, 54, 55
  down-beat, 2, 65
  vestibular, 30, 36
  latent, 2
  pelvic, 25
  pendular, 1, 55
  periodic alternating, 3
  pseudojerk, 55
  pseudopendular, 55
  sinusoidal, 55
  triangular, 59
  rotational, 52
  vertical monocular, 2
  vestibular, 94
Oculomotor nerve, 121
Oculomotor nucleus, 52
  horseradish peroxidase studies,
    121
  vestibular projection to, 155

Opsoclonus, 45
Optic tract
  accessory, 67
  nucleus, 67
Optokinetic afternystagmus,
    86, 93
  integrator, 97
  and labyrinthectomy, 102
Optokinetic nystagmus, 52, 77,
    86, 93, et. seq.
  and parietal lobe lesion, 5
  test, 54
Oscillopsia, 60, 67
Paramedian pontine reticular
    formation (PPRF), 42, 51,
    52
  pulse generator, 60
Perihypoglossal complex, 145
    et. seq.
Prisms, 65, 66, 67, 79
Pulse-step, 52, 54, 107
Purkinje cell, 67, 69
  eye velocity signal, 84
Reticular formation, medullary,
    105, 118
Reticular formation, pontine,
    105
  burst units, medium lead,
    109, 111-116
  burst units, long lead,
    116-117
  burst tonic units, 108
  cells unrelated to eye
    movement, 122
  connections, 121-122
  input from superior colliculus
    122-123
  pause units, 108, 117-118
  pulse and step, 108
  tonic units, 108, 118-120
Retinal blur, 45
Retinal image slip, 42, 67, 70,
    78, 79, 86
Saccades, corrective, 60
Saccades, normometric, 60
Spasmus nutans, 2
Streptomycin, 24

Superior colliculus, 122–123,
        179 et. seq.
    afferent input, 201–205
    anatomy, 180–185
    and eye movements, 197–201
    influence on motoneurones, 206
    lesion studies, 186–190
    response to non-visual stimuli,
        196
    response to visual stimuli,
        193–196
    stimulation studies, 190–193

Telescopic spectacles, 79, 81
Vestibular nerve, 68
Vestibular nuclei
    projection, 108, 139, 155
Vestibulo-ocular reflex, 13,
        65 et. seq., 72, 75 et. seq.
    dysmetria, 66, 68
    gain, 66, 67, 70, 72, 77, 79
    plasticity, 66, 68, 70, 72, 77,
        79

INDEX